MINDFULNESS

@

WORK

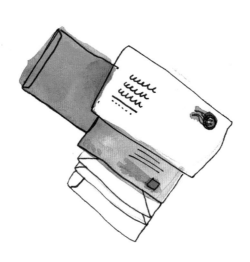

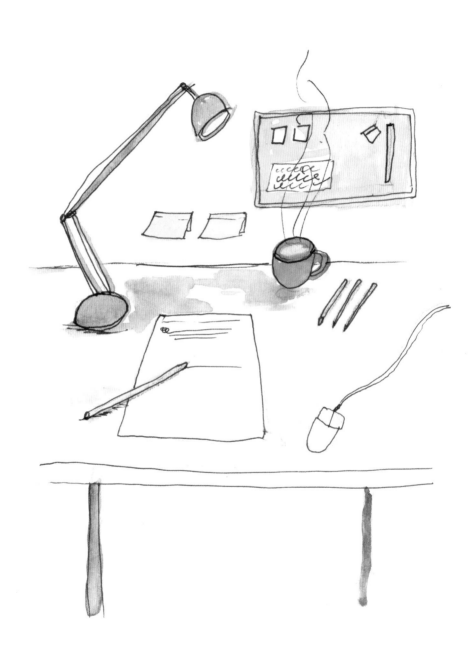

MINDFULNESS @ WORK

Reduce stress, live in the moment, and be happier and more productive at work

ANNA BLACK

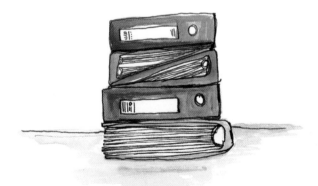

CICO BOOKS

LONDON NEW YORK

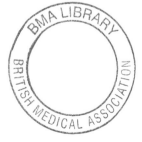

For Catherine, with thanks for your continuing friendship, wisdom, and support.

Published in 2014 by CICO Books
An imprint of Ryland Peters & Small Ltd
20-21 Jockey's Fields   519 Broadway, 5th Floor
London WC1R 4BW   New York, NY 10012

www.rylandpeters.com

10 9 8 7 6 5 4 3 2 1

Text © Anna Black 2014
Design and illustration © CICO Books 2014

A CIP catalog record for this book is available from the Library of Congress and the British Library.

ISBN: 978 1 78249 169 9

Printed in China

Editor: Jennifer Jahn
Designer: Manisha Patel
Illustrator: Amy Louise Evans

For digital editions, visit www.cicobooks.com/apps.php

CONTENTS

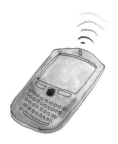

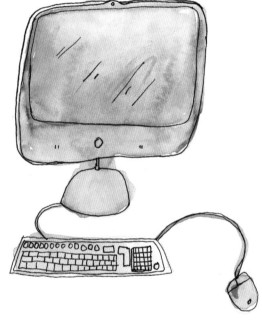

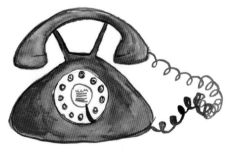

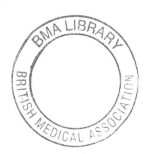

DISCOVERING MINDFULNESS

People often think meditation is not possible for them, however, mindfulness is accessible to every single one of us and chances are that you have already experienced being fully present in the moment at some point in time. Practicing mindfulness meditation is about learning how to do this intentionally—and reaping the myriad benefits.

I discovered mindfulness at a time when I was experiencing chronic stress, a good part of which was generated by work. A promotion had led to greater responsibility that, although initially exciting, became increasingly stressful as staff cuts meant that everyone was asked to do much more. A change in management caused new procedures to be implemented, and while they might have been good for the overall benefit of the company, they were less helpful for those of us who were expected to deliver them. Everyday tasks felt increasingly difficult. The more stressed we became, the more short-tempered and demanding we all grew to be; work became a place to be endured.

I was aware of the long-term health consequences of stress so I wanted to find a way to manage it. I had flirted with meditation at a local Buddhist group but I didn't want to be part of an order. I struggled with the practicalities of meditating—sitting cross-legged in lotus position was beyond me and I didn't understand what I was supposed to be doing when a teacher said to watch my mind. I had no idea how to do that so I decided that meditation must only work for certain people, and my mind must just be too busy (we always think we are special!).

By chance I stumbled across Jon Kabat-Zinn's *Full Catastrophe Living*, and this was how I first came across the term "mindfulness meditation." Reading *Full Catastrophe Living* made me realize that it was possible to establish a meditation practice outside of a spiritual framework, and I became aware of the myriad health benefits of meditation. As I began practicing mindfulness meditation, I discovered how small changes led to bigger shifts and that, if I let go of having a particular outcome in mind and instead trusted in the process, all kinds of unforeseen possibilities could emerge.

Learning to Meditate

I discovered that there was more than one way to sit while meditating and that our posture is simply a means to an end. Gradually I learned that meditation was not about stopping to think or about emptying the mind, but allowing one's thoughts to come and go without obsessing about them. I learned that my mind would always wander and that it was *repeatedly* bringing back my attention to a point of focus that was important. Over time I was able to sit still for longer periods of time. I also realized that it was not so much the length of time that was important, but rather the regularity and quality of my attention; a little and often was better than an hour once a month. I practiced tuning into my body—a place that had become unfamiliar to me over the years—and I started to notice how my body was constantly giving me accurate feedback about how I really felt. I became aware of how I would go into a meeting at work in a positive mood and how, within the space of an hour, my energy levels would plummet, my posture would change, and my neck and shoulders would become tight and stiff. I could see a direct relationship between my environment and my physical and emotional well-being.

I had assumed that a promotion was a positive thing—after all aren't we all looking for more money and greater responsibilities? Through mindfulness I learned to distinguish between what I thought was right and what I really felt and wanted at a visceral level. I realized that perhaps the responsibilities that came with the new role weren't for me as they took me further away from what I loved best about my job. When I was growing up, I had a reputation for indecisiveness. Through mindfulness and meditation I've developed trust and confidence in myself and the decisions I make—and this has been life-changing.

Accepting Our True Feelings

Acknowledging how we *really* feel, rather than how we think we should feel, is an important element of mindfulness practice. Accepting all aspects of ourselves—even the parts that we don't like or think are inappropriate—means that we are in a much stronger position to make informed decisions. We can only decide where we want to go once we have an accurate understanding of where we are right now. My mindfulness practice has taught me that nothing stays the same—I still get stressed but now I am able to recognize and so take wise action to manage it.

In my experience, practicing mindfulness at work is challenging as the workplace is often very cerebral—it is where we solve problems and fix things. The workplace is driven by goals and we have professional expectations (and people have them of us). When we feel hijacked by our emotions at work we often suppress them and distract ourselves with unhelpful strategies such as over-working, eating too much or not enough, drinking too much, or taking drugs. Or we may blow a fuse from time to time, which can create a climate of fear and uncertainty with our colleagues. We often try and apply our problem-solving skills to emotional challenges that arise but discover that what might work operationally can actually work against us emotionally, and we get caught up in unhelpful cycles of repetitive thinking or rumination.

This is a book for individuals wanting to learn about mindfulness in the workplace, rather than a guide for introducing mindfulness training into the workplace (but you can find further reading about this on page 141). I hope you will experiment with some of the more formal practices on pages 110-134 as these will help you cultivate valuable skills for applying mindfulness in the workplace. This book can only give you a taster of the possibilities that mindfulness meditation can bring into your own work and home life. If you find the practices here useful, I would encourage you to explore the subject further. There are suggestions on page 140 on how you can go about this.

MAKING THE MOST OF MINDFULNESS @ WORK

Any activity can be done mindfully — more often, the challenge is remembering to do so, particularly when we get caught up in the distractions of daily life. To help remind us and to make mindfulness an intrinsic part of our life, it is helpful to set aside a short period of time as often as you can when you can simply be with yourself—watching the breath (see page 102) or doing any of the other practices in this book. The attitudes and skills we cultivate through regular practice provide a foundation that gives us the steadiness and confidence to practice mindfulness when we are caught up in the challenges of everyday life. It is one thing to remain calm when watching the breath at home, but quite another when faced with a crisis at work or a customer losing their temper with us.

Acknowledging that what we are doing is difficult is important. We are working to change patterns of behavior that have been laid down over many years, with repeated activation. The only way we can reverse these patterns is to counteract them with multiple small actions that are positive, and thus we lay down new pathways of thinking and behavior. However, it is never a consistent path of improvement but, rather, one of ups and downs, switchbacks and fits and starts, and it's important to realize that that's okay. **It really is the journey that is the process.** It is a journey that requires patience as well as huge dollops of gentleness and kindness towards yourself. Let go of any goals to be a particular way and simply have the intention to practice as best as you can, when you can. That is all you can ask of yourself.

I recommend reading **Living in the Moment @ Work** (page 12) to find out more about stress and how it affects you and then move on to the two main sections of the book, which include practices and suggestions for bringing mindfulness into the workplace: **You @ Work** (see page 44) and **You and Others @ Work** (see page 80), and because how we are at work affects how we behave at home, there is also a section on **@ Home** (see page 100). I strongly recommend that you try some of the more "formal" practices in the @ Home chapter, as the skills cultivated will stand you in good stead in helping you to apply mindfulness to your day-to-day working life.

You can read from cover to cover or randomly choose a practice to try. If the practices resonate with you, you may find yourself gradually incorporating more and more of them into your daily life. Be creative about how you apply mindfulness to your work; many of the practices here could easily be adapted to different scenarios, so don't assume that there is only one way to do something.

If you are interested, explore the subject further with the suggestions on **Where to Go Next** (page 140) and **Further Reading** (page 141)

Do It Your Way

The practices are predominantly informal practices and they are a good place to start if you are a beginner. If you have an adverse reaction to any of the practices please stop and get advice from a mindfulness teacher or healthcare professional before continuing.

If you already have some experience with mindfulness meditation, I hope this book will encourage you to bring it more into your work life. The more we can weave mindfulness into the fabric of our daily life, the more we will reap the benefits.

CHAPTER ONE

LIVING IN THE MOMENT @ WORK

Stress at work is a leading cause of absenteeism and can have long-term health consequences. This chapter looks at stress, how it affects us, and how regularly practicing mindfulness can help, both physiologically and psychologically. When we feel well, we are more likely to perform at our best.

Through regularly practicing mindfulness meditation we become used to noticing what we are feeling in the head, heart, and body. This awareness can cultivate a pause that is long enough for us to stop and stand back, thereby turning an automatic reaction into a considered response, which can have a valuable practical application:

"It was the last day before the holidays and I had been exchanging e-mails with a client who, I thought, was being needlessly obstructive about something I'd been hoping to finalize that day. As I typed a reply to him I was aware of how annoyed I was—I could feel it in the way I hammered the keyboard! Noticing this was enough to make me pause—I knew I was angry, so I decided to do nothing for the time being and deleted my intended reply. A few hours later I had an email from the client conceding that their original request was unnecessary and I could go ahead as I had originally suggested. I was pleased that I had used my mindfulness practice to notice how I was reacting and so to pause and reflect, and stop the situation from escalating and potentially damaging my relationship with the client."

Alex's awareness of what was happening in her body as well as of the rising irritation and frustration had been cultivated through regularly practicing mindfulness. Her awareness acted like a red flag,and giving her the ability to stop and pause. Rather than react impulsively and potentially damage a relationship, she responded differently, resulting in a positive outcome for all concerned. This is just one example of how regular mindfulness practice influences our behavior.

MINDFULNESS IN THE WORKPLACE

The "workplace" can take different forms—for many of us it is an office, but for you the workplace could also be a hospital or clinic, a school or college, a prison or law enforcement agency, a shop, a supermarket, or an establishment in the service industry. You might work at a desk or in the outdoors, within a team of people or perhaps remotely from home, interacting rarely with others. You might go to the same place every day for years or your workplace may be changing all the time; you may work on land, sea, or in the air. Whatever you do and wherever you do it, the bottom line is that the workplace is where all of us spend the majority of time as adults and, regardless of whether we enjoy it or not, we work to earn a living and contribute to society. When we meet new people one of the first bits of information we often share is what we do professionally. Work gives us an identity and often a particular status in society. This is significant because if our identity is defined by what we do, and we spend the majority of our waking life at work, when something goes wrong or becomes challenging in our work environment, the effect on us can be devastating.

Evidence suggests that many of us find the workplace challenging. The Health and Safety Executive in the UK reports that one in five employees feels very or extremely stressed at work (that's the equivalent of five million people in the UK). Work-induced stress is now the most common reason for-long term sickness absence. The cost of this is estimated to be £3.7 billion per year. In the USA, the National Institute for Occupational Safety and Health reports that stress-related ailments cost companies $200 billion per year, with 70–90 percent of hospital visits by employees linked to stress.

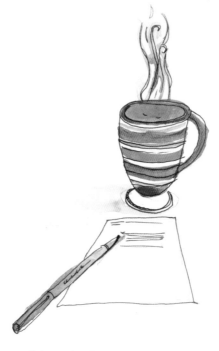

A 2010 report on mindfulness by the UK's Mental Health Foundation includes survey results showing that:

- 81% of those surveyed agree that "the fast pace of life and the number of things we have to do and worry about these days is a major cause of stress, unhappiness and illness in UK society;"

- 86% agree that "people would be much happier and healthier if they knew how to slow down and live in the moment;"

- 53% agree that "I find it difficult to relax or switch off, and can't stop myself thinking about things I have to do or nagging worries."

But how can we learn to switch off? How can we slow down and avoid getting swept up in the fast-paced world of work and home-life? How do we balance "living in the moment" with making sure that we are looking after our family's future? One way we can do this is by practicing mindfulness meditation, through which we can cultivate and learn these skills.

WHAT IS MINDFULNESS?

Mindfulness is a term that is frequently used in the media but there are often misconceptions about what it actually means. Mindfulness is commonly defined as: Deliberately paying attention to your experience as it arises without judgment.

The key elements are:

- **Intentionality**—we are *deliberately* paying attention.

- We are **noticing in a particular way**, *without judging our experience*, that it is what it is, and that there is no right or wrong.

- We are doing this **moment by moment**—noticing how our experience is constantly changing. Our experience encompasses **thoughts, physical sensations, and emotions.**

Paying Attention

It is important that we pay attention in this specific way because our regular activities are often done on autopilot. We perform habitual actions, such as locking up the house or traveling to work, without even being aware of it, and if we were asked to recount the action/event we are often unable to do so. To a certain extent we need to operate that way to get as many things done in the time we do have. However, problems arise when we spend the majority of our life on autopilot, when zoning out becomes our default. Our lack of attention means that we don't notice something or we miss things that are going on, and this affects our relationships with others. We multi-task to the extent that we never stop and just take stock of where we are. Or we might be stuck; paralyzed with thoughts of "what if" or "if only" that prevent us from moving forward and dealing with what is going on now. The negativity that arises out of these states of mind affects us even further and we end up working harder. We may become anxious, depressed, or begin to self-medicate with drugs and alcohol, and so the vicious cycle continues.

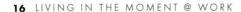

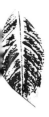

Very often this cycle is only broken by some major life change, such as an illness or accident, a bereavement or a relationship breakdown that jolts us awake and makes us question the way we live. In the workplace this type of breakdown is sometimes called a "burnout" and on pages 22–37 we look at how stress can cause a burnout and how mindfulness can help prevent it.

Origins of Mindfulness

Cultivating mindfulness through meditation is nothing new and its origins can be found in Buddhist practices that are over 2,500 years old.

In 1979 mindfulness began to be used therapeutically by Dr. Jon Kabat-Zinn and colleagues at the Stress Reduction Clinic at the University of Massachusetts Hospital, USA. Kabat-Zinn developed the 8-week Mindfulness-Based Stress Reduction (MBSR) program as a way of helping people learn to live with chronic medical conditions. The MBSR program uses both formal (e.g. sitting, the body scan, and movement practices) and informal meditation practices and helps participants cultivate qualities such as patience, acceptance, and equanimity.

In 2001 Mindfulness-Based Cognitive Therapy (MBCT) was developed by Mark Williams, John Teasdale, and Zindel V. Segal. Based on MBSR, MBCT was developed specifically for the treatment of depression, but has since been adapted in the treatment of many other conditions, including anxiety, eating disorders, and addiction. MBCT is recommended by the National Institute of Clinical Excellence (NICE) in the UK for the treatment of depression in individuals who have suffered three or more episodes.

In essence, MBSR and MBCT are very similar. MBSR is usually taught to generic groups of people suffering from a variety of physical and psychological conditions and/or general life stress, while MBCT is usually taught to a group of people suffering from a specific condition such as depression or anxiety. The emphasis on deliberate and non-judgmental present-moment awareness of one's own experience is at the core of both programs.

Benefits of Mindfulness

As the evidence base for the therapeutic uses of mindfulness-based approaches to health is growing all the time, the wider applications of mindfulness continue to be explored. Today there are mindfulness programs in schools, prisons, in sports as well as healthcare, and it is practiced as much by healthcare providers as by patients themselves. In addition, there is an entire area of mindfulness in the workplace in which we are interested here.

The evidence for the benefits of mindfulness at work is compelling. Participants in MBSR workplace programs report the following:

- being more engaged in their work;

- feeling more energized and less anxious after the course;

- experiencing fewer medical symptoms and less psychological distress;

- being able to concentrate better

(Mental Health Foundation Report on Mindfulness 2010)

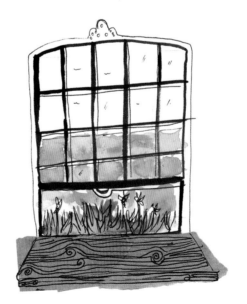

Studies carried out on the effectiveness of mindfulness training in the workplace have shown positive benefits on both a personal and business level. In Britain, Transport for London (TfL) employees who received mindfulness-based training reported improvements in their relationships (80%), in the ability to relax (79%), in their sleep patterns (64%), and in happiness at work (53%). These improvements continued long after the course had finished. Absenteeism due to stress, anxiety, and depression fell by 71% over the following three years.

> *"Participants learn that they have some control over their responses even if they can't control the events themselves—what a customer says to them for example."*

Emerald-Jane Turner, Developer of TfL course

(Mental Health Foundation Mindfulness Report, 2010).

In the USA, a detachment of US marines received an adapted mindfulness program (Mindfulness-based Mind Fitness Training) to help them deal more effectively with the stress of active duty. The study showed a correlation between practice time and increased mindfulness, which in turn was associated with a decrease in their perceived stress. Individually, marines reported benefits such as the ability to stay focused, to stay with difficult experiences, to work with difficult emotions and unhealthy coping strategies, as well as reporting improvements in family life. Leaders reported an improved ability to recognize emotions in themselves and others, which enabled them to be more receptive to feedback. They also reported a better understanding of their strengths and weaknesses and were better able to identify early warning signs of stress. As a group, they noted improved team communication and a greater sense of cohesiveness. Overall they felt that the group was more in control of chaotic situations.

Many of the benefits reported in general mindfulness groups, i.e. not carried out specifically in workplace programs, are equally relevant for the work environment.

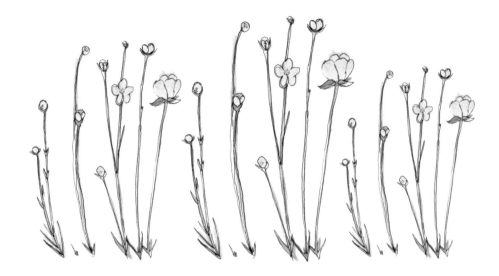

Meditation Changes the Brain

Practicing mindfulness meditation can also result in physiological changes. Neuroscientists have shown that it can cause a shift in activity from the right to the left prefrontal cortex, which is associated with more positive emotions and the ability to handle difficult emotions. They also discovered differences in the brains of practitioners in the areas associated with decision-making, attention, and awareness. Regular meditation can also result in increased brain size in areas linked to emotion regulation, boost the immune system, and lower blood pressure.

There is also a proven correlation between mindfulness and emotional intelligence. Emotional intelligence is associated with good social skills, and the ability to cooperate with others and see the bigger picture. The most successful business leaders are those with a high degree of emotional intelligence.

It is important to note that the research is commonly conducted on people learning mindfulness meditation on a structured course lasting six to eight weeks, and which includes daily formal practices such as sitting, the body scan, and mindful movement, as well as more informal practices, during which participants are encouraged to practice mindfulness in their everyday environment.

REPORTED BENEFITS

- Increased ability to focus and concentrate
- More positive relationships
- Improved personal efficiency and productivity
- Improved ability to handle stress
- Better able to listen
- Better able to think and respond more creatively
- Healthier life/work balance
- Better able to manage staff
- More thoughtful and deliberate decision-making
- Improved physical and mental well-being
- Greater awareness of social dynamics

- Better able to set aside a personal agenda
- Improved empathy
- Improved memory (particularly in a stressful environment)
- Better able to let go of judgments
- Ability to see a broader perspective
- Improved emotional stability
- Decrease in anger
- Increased positive outlook
- Better able to handle difficult emotions
- Reduced anxiety
- Reduced depression
- More energetic
- More engaged with work

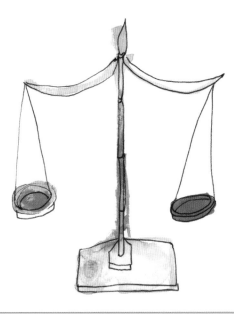

MINDFULNESS AND STRESS

It is important to acknowledge that even when we do practice mindfulness we will experience stress—**stress is the body's natural and essential warning signal** to us to say "Enough! You are at risk." There will still be occasions when you get swept away by what is going on in your life; this happens to us all. It doesn't mean that you have failed or that mindfulness has failed. It is just another opportunity to recognize the edge along which we all balance as we live life. When I experienced a period of chronic stress, with the benefit of mindfulness, I was able to notice how it affected me physically and psychologically.

Life is stressful and particularly the workplace where so much is out of our control. There will always be periods of difficulty. We will never "get it," we are always practicing, learning, and growing—and that is okay. An image that may be useful is that of a ball rolling down a hill, going faster and faster as it gathers momentum. Mindfulness is like a hand that reaches out and stops the ball momentarily. The ball may start rolling again, but that check has slowed it down. **Mindfulness offers us those moments that can prevent things from spiraling out of control**. Those moments provide an opportunity to make a single small change that can have a much bigger effect in the long run.

Work Stress

Chronic stress creeps up on us unexpectedly. Perhaps a colleague is sick or the economic downturn means a freeze on hiring or even redundancies, and we are asked to pick up the slack. Maybe there is a change in management and consequently a shift in culture and what is expected of us. Perhaps we get a promotion that brings with it new responsibilities and expectations. Whatever the particular circumstance might be, there is a change that affects us.

Chronic Stress: A Personal Account

It is accepted that increased pressure can improve our performance—but only to a certain point. If the pressure rises too much, our ability to cope and thrive falls away and we begin to become stressed and possibly even ill. There will come a point for everyone when, instead of enhancing performance, increasing pressure will start to undermine it.

Even a simple paper jam in the printer could incur my wrath and I noticed how quickly negativity spread from colleague to colleague.

This happened to me. I observed how, over a period of time, my personality changed as I was expected to take on an increasing workload. I became short-tempered and much less tolerant of others, particularly those whom I felt were stopping me from moving forward with a particular task. I would keep particular storylines alive outside of work as I would share them with friends and family. I noticed how, while recounting earlier events, those negative thoughts would have a direct impact on my body—I could feel the mounting tension, particularly in my shoulders and neck. My voice would take on a particular tone and my breathing become more rapid. I noticed, too, how I would select events that corroborated the story I was telling—discounting any others that might have made the situation more balanced. I noticed how I became prone to catastrophizing. I became forgetful and found it difficult to concentrate. I was less focused than usual and would jump from task to task as I felt overwhelmed with the work at hand; sometimes I would feel paralyzed and stuck —with so much to do, where to start? Unusually for me I became prone to tears and even panic attacks. I lost a sense of perspective and my perception of events at work became either black or white.

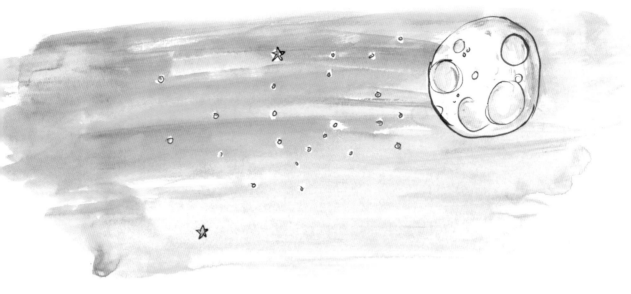

I noticed how my anxiety spread outside of work. My normally good sleep patterns became disrupted as I'd wake up in the night thinking about work. I began breaking my own rules and repeatedly checked my work emails in the evenings and over the weekend. This constantly pulled me into thinking about work rather than allowing me to mentally take time off from work pressures. I started going into work earlier and earlier so I could finish tasks, which meant that there was no possibility to fit in a yoga class or other exercise beforehand. I took the bus rather than walk as that would get me to work 15 minutes earlier. At the end of the day and work week, I was too tired to do many of the things that would usually nourish me and so I would vegetate in front of the television.

When the more intense periods of stress had eased off again, I discovered that the habits I had fallen into had become the norm. I became aware of how much I was contributing to and stoking my own stress.

My experience was a classic case of **chronic stress—the repeated activation of the body's stress response**. The stress response is automatic and unconscious, so usually it happens below our radar. It can helpful to know what is actually going on in the body when the stress response is activated, and what maintains it, so that we can take steps to break the cycle.

WHAT IS STRESS?

It is important to remember that we would not be able to survive without the body's built-in reaction to stress. This function is located in the most primitive part of the brain and it is this that has kept Homo sapiens alive over millennia and continues to do so today. The stress reaction is the body's instant and well-oiled response to a threat that alerts us to danger and causes us to react instantly. In times of danger people often report being able to draw on seemingly impossible reserves of strength or speed to save themselves or someone else. This is a result of the body's tremendous capacity to respond effectively to danger. If we were unable to experience the stress response we would die.

The body's response to stress can also be useful to us at other times. As we will see overleaf, when we are nervous, the body gives us very specific signals to alert us when something different to the norm is happening. We literally "wake up" in the present moment. The release of adrenaline before a presentation, crucial meeting, or decision-making can give us an important edge. We are hypersensitive to what is going on as our senses are on high alert and we can respond accordingly. People often report that being on this "edge" is beneficial.

The problem arises when the body's stress reaction is out of kilter, when it becomes over-active and responds to events, thoughts, or feelings that are perceived as life threatening when in reality they are not. The key word here is **perceived**.

The way we see, interpret, and evaluate what is happening around us is crucial —and will differ for each one of us. **If we can change the way we perceive what is happening, we can change our experience of it**. The good news is that mindfulness meditation is a particularly effective way of relating to our experience in a different manner, thereby changing our perception of it and reducing its threat.

The Stress Response in Action

The body radar is on constant alert for any perceived threat, external or internal. Our senses are continuously taking in external information and can trigger an alarm. This alarm can also be set off by an internal threat—a thought, emotion, or physical pain. Whatever the trigger, the alarm activates an instantaneous response in parts of the brain, including the amygdala. This activation sets off a chain reaction (see right).

All of these physical changes will increase our chance of survival if the threat we are facing is an external one. When we literally "fight" or "flee" in response to danger, the stress hormones that are causing all these physical changes are dispersed and the body returns to balance or homeostasis. This is how it should be.

While the body reacts to a threat, the brain continues to gather information from external sources through the senses, but also by accessing the higher centers of the brain—our thoughts, experiences, memories, knowledge, etc., in order to determine the degree of threat and whether the alert should be maintained or deactivated. **Problems occur when the body's alarm is constantly being activated for perceived threats that pose no real danger.** These might be an angry exchange with a colleague or customer, a paper jam in the photocopier, a deadline brought forward, being late for a meeting... **The more often the stress response is activated, the more sensitive it becomes**. The body moves into a state of hyper-arousal and such repeated activation creates chronic stress. The stress hormones never have the chance to be dispersed through natural means and they play havoc with the body, both physically and emotionally.

THE BODY'S RESPONSE TO STRESS

★ Release of hormones, such as glucocorticoids and cortisol, which produce a range of different stress responses.

★ Release of chemical messengers, including dopamine, norepinephrine or epinephrine, also known as adrenaline. These neurotransmitters suppress activity in the front area of the brain, thus negatively affecting short-term memory, concentration, inhibition, and rational thinking. They also interfere with our ability to handle difficult social or intellectual tasks and behaviors. The role of these stress hormones is to make the body ready for fight or flight—two actions crucial for survival—and we feel the physical effect immediately.

★ The heart begins to pump much faster. The rate of blood flow may increase by 300–400 percent in order to get blood around the body more quickly, particularly to the arms or legs (for fighting or fleeing).

★ The skin may become cold and clammy as blood is diverted to support the heart and muscles and reduce blood loss in case of injury.

★ Pupils may dilate to improve sight.

★ Body hair may stand on end to sense vibrations and/or danger.

★ The mouth may become dry as fluid is diverted from non-essential locations. The throat may spasm.

★ Non-essential body functions are shut down as the body's priority is survival. Butterflies in the stomach signify digestion shutting down. There is often a need to go to the toilet to evacuate any unnecessary weight to aid flight. Reproductive organs are shut down as perpetuating the species is immaterial if death is imminent.

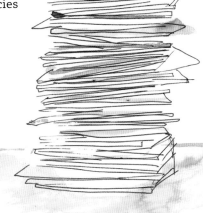

This is what is happening to us every time we feel stressed—often several times a day.

CHRONIC STRESS

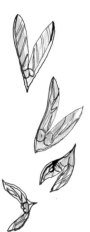

The repeated activation of the stress reaction puts the body under constant physical stress. The increase in blood pressure raises the risk of heart disease while the presence of stress hormones interferes with insulin activity, thereby increasing the risk of diabetes. The immune system is disrupted, making us more vulnerable to illness and disease. Chronic stress equals constant stress; this means that there is no natural dispersal of stress hormones so they remain in the body causing havoc:

- The release of cortisol is toxic in the long term. It causes the amygdala to become overactive, creating fearful thinking and negativity, and thus a feedback loop that maintains stress. The function of the higher center of the brain that overrides the on-switch of the stress reaction becomes inhibited and disrupted, so the calming response (see page 30) is impaired.

- Cortisol affects neural branching in the brain and inhibits the building of new neurons so that we get stuck in old patterns of fearful thinking. It also causes atrophy in the area of the brain where new brain cells are produced. So, the possibility of developing new ways of thinking is diminished.

- The functions of the prefrontal cortex, such as memory, decision-making, and thought processes are disrupted; concentration is impaired.

- Depression is caused or worsened by the depletion of serotonin.

- The long-term functions of the body, such as digestion and reproduction, are repeatedly disrupted, affecting functionality.

- Mood swings increase, along with general anxiety and even panic.

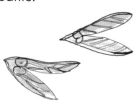

Long-term effects of chronic stress may include fatigue, lack of energy and motivation, disruption to sleep patterns, autoimmune disorders, fertility, and digestive problems. We often adopt coping strategies to deal with these unpleasant side-effects. We are not as effective as usual, so we may work harder and longer or we may use work to serve as a distraction. Perhaps we take work home with us or stay connected 24/7 via our phones and tablets. We may drink more and medicate with prescription or recreational drugs. Or we may skip meals, overeat, or eat unhealthily because we don't have time to shop and cook. These strategies may appear to be helpful and they can often help in the short term. If we are young and fit, it may take time for us to become aware of the consequences, but **sooner or later stress catches up with all of us.**

Chronic stress is a vicious circle as it strengthens negative networks and weakens the positive ones. We may find ourselves giving up that evening class or choir practice, not going for that walk or to the gym, turning down an invitation to socialize with friends because we are too tired. As we try and stay on top of things—by giving up what we think of as the "extras"—our world can quickly become narrower and narrower and more work-focused. We may feel as if our life lacks meaning but we don't know how to make it better so we become frustrated and dissatisfied.

If work occupies the majority of our time (both physically and mentally), when something does go wrong, it may feel as if our entire life is falling apart because we don't have enough going on outside of work to balance it. Our identity is completely wrapped up in who we are at work and when that is challenged we are shaken to our very core. So what options are available to recover from or prevent this from happening? Just as our body has an in-built stress reaction, it also has a corresponding calming response that operates in the same automatic and unconscious manner. However, the calming response can also be activated deliberately, and regularly practicing mindfulness can help us do that.

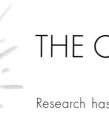

THE CALMING RESPONSE

Research has shown that the brain is much more plastic and malleable than previously thought. This means that there is real potential to change the way we think and act, and each one of us can influence that through our behavior.

In addition to the cognitive memory that we are all familiar with, we also have a body memory. The body retains a response to a particular thought or action and activates this same reaction automatically whenever it arises. This is why, when the body perceives something as a threat, it may continue activating the stress reaction even though the threat is long past its sell-by date. However, the positive side of this means that it is possible to learn a different way of responding to a situation and thereby creating new body memories. We can do this with mindfulness, bearing in mind that it takes time, patience, and kindness towards ourselves.

Practicing mindfulness is one way of deliberately activating the calming response —the body's built-in off-switch for the stress-reaction cycle. The body's stress reaction is automatic and unconscious. Turning the lens of awareness onto what is happening during this reaction will, by its very nature, change it. When we bring an attitude of acknowledgment and curiosity to our experiences, we are immediately taking a different stance—witnessing what is unfolding as we are observing rather than being caught up in the experience. This immediately has a dampening effect on any emotional charge. This moment of conscious awareness removes us from reacting unconsciously, thereby creating an opportunity for choice. As feelings of stress are often characterized by experiencing a lack of control, the introduction of choice immediately increases a sense of being incontrol. We can now decide how to respond next. This will reduce the stress we are feeling. When we respond mindfully not only do we experience a personal benefit, but the change in behavior is likely to prevent or nip in the bud a negative chain reaction from occurring in our dealings with others.

When we regularly practice letting go of thoughts and returning to a point of focus, such as the breath in sitting practice (see page 102), we are strengthening these neural pathways and creating a body memory for "this is what we do with sticky thoughts." Thus, when we bring awareness to anxious thoughts arising due to stress, using the breath as an anchor will become a familiar feeling, letting go and bringing ourselves back again and again prevents us from getting stuck in rumination; it will also help reduce the activation of fearful thoughts that can keep the stress-reaction cycle activated. Creating a pause in this way is creating an opportunity for the higher areas of the brain to contextualize the perceived threat, gather more information from the senses, memories, and experiences, and thereby deactivate the emergency signal.

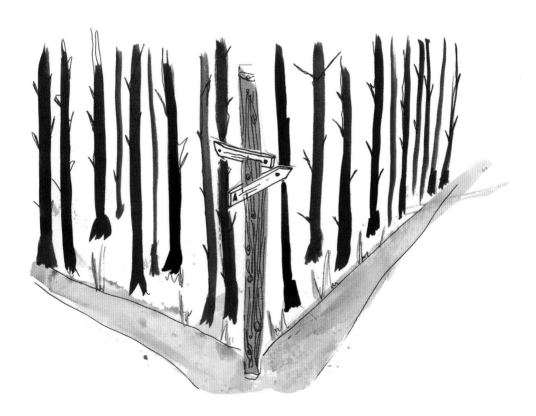

KEEPING CALM WITH MINDFULNESS

Although it is never too late to work on our stress management, it is much easier to build up our stress hardiness during periods when we are not actually experiencing chronic stress. Not only is it easier to learn new skills and establish healthy routines when we are feeling well, but these skills will also help us spot warning signs much earlier and enable us to be better equipped to handle stress when it does arise. As Jon Kabat-Zinn often says, you want to weave your parachute before you need it.

Remember that stress is often caused by feeling a lack of control. Our mindfulness practice highlights how our experience is constantly changing and, as we become familiar and therefore more comfortable with change and the lack of control this brings, it helps us feel more confident handling it. If we can learn to adapt to change we will be better equipped to manage stress.

Learning from Experience

When we practice mindfulness regularly, we become aware of our habitual thoughts and behaviors; we become familiar with our breathing and how it changes under stress; we are in tune with the body and its arising physical sensations. Perhaps we notice that what we thought was anger was, in reality, fear, and we learn to recognize what fear actually feels like physically. When we are familiar with something, we don't perceive it as threatening.

Regular practice of mindfulness also helps create a greater awareness of the bigger picture—how our biases and habitual stories that we bring to situations can feed our anxiety. Through our practice we become familiar with the holes we regularly fall into because of our negative thinking, and so we help establish a greater chance of recognizing our own contribution to the situation.

Mindfulness thus creates a familiarity with our own experiences, whether they are negative, positive, or neutral. Mindfulness enables us to create our very own early warning system and we become much more likely to pick up on small changes that signal that the body is under stress. It might be noticing a particular thought tone (see page 52), or becoming aware of the physical undercurrent of anxiety, or changes in our eating or sleeping—but awareness of such change signals us to take wise action.

It is important to note that practicing mindfulness does not stop us from feeling emotions. My own experience supports research finding that meditators do experience negative feelings and stress, and that they can actually feel them more strongly than non-meditators. However, they recover from such feelings more quickly. By letting go of difficult thoughts and emotions they don't get stuck in the same way as non-meditators may do.

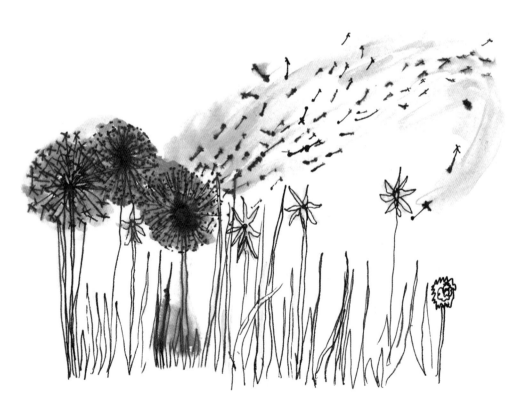

ACTIVATING THE CALMING RESPONSE

The body has its own automatic activation of the calming response. As the body/mind assesses the perceived threat, information is gathered from the senses and the higher centers of the brain that will maintain or deactivate the stress response.

However, we can also deliberately activate the calming response: **first we must acknowledge what is actually happening**. Acknowledgment means allowing oneself to become aware of the experience—noticing the thoughts, emotions, and physical sensations arising (even if we don't like them, want them, or think they are inappropriate). The act of acknowledgment is crucial and must not be underestimated or ignored. Acknowledgment is the first step towards acceptance or being with our experience, which is the essence of the transformative power of mindfulness. Simply bringing awareness to the body and noticing the tension in the shoulders or jaw, for example, will often result in an instant softening or letting go.

Bringing an attitude of curious awareness to your experience (specifically what is arising in the body) will break the constant mulling over of thoughts that is rumination. The brain can't be interested in the present experience and at the same time be stuck in the past or the future—so awareness of the body brings about an immediate shift to the present moment. This creates the opportunity for the higher centers of the brain to do their job—that is to contextualize and interpret what is happening without negative bias.

You might also want to **use the breath or "feet on floor" as an anchor to the present moment** (see pages 54, 78, and 47), and so engage the calming response.

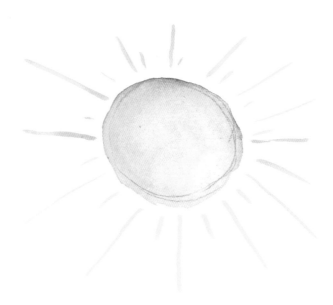

When the calming response is activated, the body responds accordingly (the threat is removed so there is no need to prime the body for fight or flight):

- The heart rate slows down.

- Blood pressure falls.

- Breathing slows and settles to its normal rate.

- Muscles soften and relax as tension is released.

The more often we can deliberately activate the calming response, the more familiar it will become to the body. The body will learn and remember that *this* is what it does when a similar situation arises in the future. This is important as it means that the **more we practice mindfulness, the more we are creating and storing new patterns of learned behavior**—positive ones, rather than the negative ones created by chronic stress.

BUILD EMOTIONAL RESILIENCE

Research has shown that if we practice mindfulness regularly—even when we are not stressed—we are building up emotional resilience or stress hardiness, which will stand us in good stead when we are stressed. When we feel stressed we often feel a lack of control or choice. However, mindfulness gives us choice, and choice gives us options. Someone who has developed stress hardiness will:

- View life as a challenge.

- Assume an active role in attempting to exert meaningful control over life.

- Have a strong internal conviction that they are able to manage whatever life throws at them.

Cultivate Awareness

Developing awareness through mindfulness highlights the links between our environment, lifestyle, and what we are experiencing. We eat a donut or candy and notice an immediate rush of energy, but we also become aware of the crash in mood a couple of hours later. We notice how our mood is affected after a "gossiping session" around the watercooler about how bad everything is. We notice how our child withdraws from us when we pretend to listen to their latest discovery while we are actually reading our work e-mail. We become aware of the whole picture and can **contextualize our experience**. We acknowledge our own biases and judgments without condemnation, but are taking them into account—we notice small details about colleagues and their behavior and body language. This additional knowledge gives us feedback and informs the way we interact with them.

We become aware of our own habitual patterns of thoughts and behaviors and more tuned into our experience and so are better able to take wise action.

Mindfulness can help us deal with stressful situations in the moment and thus prevent intermittent stress from developing into chronic stress, with all the negative health and performance issues that it brings. Mindfulness can also help us build up our stress hardiness so that we are better able to weather the storms when they do come. Mindfulness also helps cultivate positive changes in the way we connect with others by developing compassion, empathy, and greater flexibility in relationships; it causes physiological changes in the brain, particularly in the so-called executive functions, improving attention, focus, and concentration, as well as positive emotions.

Mindfulness cultivates an approach—rather than avoidance —mode of thinking and this, in turn, has been shown to improve creative thinking. In avoidance mode our thinking becomes much narrower and more blinkered. Mindfulness encourages acceptance—acceptance of ourselves and of others, which frees us from the tyranny of perfectionism and the need for things to be a particular way. Mindfulness helps us notice how much is good in our life, and so even in difficult circumstances we are aware of and can benefit from the lightness and richness that is around and has the potential to nourish us if we allow it.

All of these benefits and more have a bearing in the workplace on us as individuals, as well as on what we contribute through our performance and interaction with colleagues, clients, or customers.

COMMON MISCONCEPTIONS

People often have concerns about meditation or perhaps have heard about different techniques, so it is helpful to answer some frequently asked questions here.

How can mindfulness help so many different conditions—both physical and psychological?

Mindfulness is not a quick fix or magic bullet that will cure all ills. The evidence base suggests that it can be helpful with a wide range of physical and psychological conditions. While there are proven physical benefits (see page 21), mindfulness also helps us relate to whatever may be going on in our lives in a different way and this then has a positive effect on symptoms. However, practicing mindfulness meditation does require a commitment and willingness to be with whatever arises, and this can be challenging.

I can't stop thinking—my mind is too busy to meditate.

We are not trying to empty or clear our mind when we meditate. Instead, we are observing our thoughts and noticing common patterns or stories. Generally, we are unaware of the stories that are influencing and driving all our actions and decisions. By bringing them into awareness we are in a better position to discard those that aren't helpful and deliberately encourage those that are. As we become familiar with our particular stories or judgments, we are able to take into account these biases in our interactions with others.

Does mindfulness conflict with religion?

Mindfulness meditation is totally secular. Its origins are in ancient Buddhist practices but practicing mindfulness meditation should not conflict with any existing religious practice you have, and you can practice mindfulness without subscribing to any religious beliefs.

Will mindfulness help me relax?

We are not meditating in order to relax or, indeed, to achieve any particular state of mind. We may become more relaxed as a result of meditation but if we set out to become relaxed by meditating, we are setting ourselves up for failure and disappointment. When we meditate we are opening ourselves up to whatever arises. All mind states and emotions will arise at some point when we do formal practices, and this presents us with opportunities to be with difficult emotions in a safe environment. In this way we can cultivate skills that we can then put into practice when difficult emotions arise in everyday life. However, as we come to realize that much of our unhappiness is caused by our thoughts and the way we relate to them, and as we learn new ways to deal with this, we find ourselves feeling calmer and less stressed.

Is mindfulness just positive thinking?

Mindfulness is not positive thinking. We are not trying to convince ourselves that everything is wonderful in the world. On the contrary, mindfulness is about opening up to all experiences: the positive, the negative, and the neutral. Each is as worthy of our attention as the other. We need to acknowledge and experience the dark as well as the light, and all of the shades of gray in between. Through opening up to the full spectrum, we begin to see how circumstances change and states of mind ebb and flow like the tide, and that nothing is fixed forever. There always exists the possibility for change; one small change often leads to another.

Isn't "living in the moment" irresponsible?

When we talk of "living in the moment" it does not mean living without any thoughts for the future. Living in the moment simply means paying attention to our experience as it happens and really knowing (and acknowledging) what is actually happening. It is only in this moment that we are better able to take care of and influence what is going to happen next. What we do in this moment will determine what happens next.

I can't sit cross-legged on the floor—does that mean I can't meditate?

We do not need to sit in a special position to meditate. It is not the position that is important but the attitude of mind we bring to it. If, for any reason, you find it difficult to do a practice as suggested, then it is always fine to adapt and change a practice to suit how you are in this moment. Pages 42–43 have more guidance on posture.

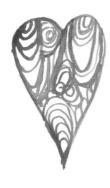

HELPFUL ATTITUDES

Practicing mindfulness regularly cultivates particular attitudes and in turn, deliberately encouraging these particular attitudes supports and deepens our practice further.

CURIOSITY is the touchstone of mindfulness practice. When we are curious about our experience we become interested in what is happening to us. This creates a sense of witnessing that prevents us from becoming embroiled in the emotion, but it also holds our attention and so the mind is less likely to wander. If we are interested in something, we want to find out more about it so we move in a little bit closer. What do you notice? Where do you notice it? What is it like? We are not interested in "why" but simply "what." When we move in closer, we engage in an approach rather than an avoidant state of mind. When we are curious, we see things as if for the first time as we drop the filters of past experience and open up to the possibilities of whatever might be there. We don't have a particular expectation or goal in mind.

If we are focused on achieving a specific result we can be blind to the myriad possibilities that might also arise and so we practice **NON–STRIVING.** When we are goal–oriented, if our experience is different to what we expected we will be disappointed and may reject the experience. Rather than focus on the end result it is helpful to continually remind ourselves that the best way to get anywhere is simply to focus on what's here right now. Whenever you notice a driven quality in your practice it is an alert—a signal to let go.

When we are pulled away by our thoughts in our practice, we let them go and return to the point of focus. This is the point of the practice and we do it over and over again to practice **LETTING GO** of the thought, the pins and needles, the emotions. It is only through letting go that we can learn to be with how things really are—whether good, bad, or indifferent. By practicing letting go of the need for things to be fixed or changed we are learning to accept things as they really are.

In mindfulness, **ACCEPTANCE** is not passive resignation but a positive active step. By ackowledging how things really are (rather than how we would like them to be) we have a clear starting place from which we can move forward. Acceptance is characterized by an approach frame of mind. We are not resisting our experience but moving toward it or simply being with it. We can do this by being curious about it. When we start practicing we are often shocked at how judgmental we actually are and how these judgments influence our thinking and behavior.

When we pay attention to our thoughts we notice the constant barrage of criticisms about ourself and others, and just being aware of this can be really helpful—noticing without adding a layer of judgments about the judging is the challenge! We practice **NON-JUDGING,** as judgments box us in and stop us from seeing the whole picture, and they are often harsh. Non-judging goes hand in hand with **KINDNESS**. By letting go of the judging mind and the mean thoughts, we are practicing kindness to ourselves and others. It is okay to have an opinion or a degree of discernment, but we are learning to see the whole context of a situation rather than just one narrow viewpoint.

It is important to **TRUST IN THE PROCESS**. This attitude ties in closely with non-striving and patience. Learning to trust in the body and your own experience and having the courage and patience to let things unfold in their own time will grow with your mindfulness practice and so we learn to access and trust in our own inner wisdom.

Mindfulness is not a quick fix. We may feel some benefits quite quickly but long-term transformational change takes time, and often other people may notice how you have changed before you do. Let go of measuring how you are improving (or not) and through practicing watching the breath and "being with the itch", we learn **PATIENCE** and the ability to stay.

It is important to remember that we are all works in progress—we don't need to be a paragon of virtue to practice mindfulness. There is never a perfect time to do something and too often we put things off because of this—we simply start from where we are, however that is. Regularly doing the formal practices on pages 100–139 will help cultivate these attitudes and each one supports the other. When you notice how impatient or judgmental you are or how you are disappointed when something didn't turn out as you had expected, don't give yourself a hard time. Simply acknowledge and name it and be gentle with yourself. Mindfulness is not about judgments or evaluation but rather a personal journey of discovery and self-enlightenment.

SITTING COMFORTABLY

It is a common misconception that to meditate means that we have to sit like a pretzel in lotus position—something that is beyond the reach of the majority of us. However, **we can meditate in a variety of different positions and no one is better than another. The pose is simply a means to an end.**

Many of the practices in this book are going to be done when you are out and about at work. You may be sitting behind a desk or at a counter; you may be spending most of your time on your feet, and so it is not going to be possible to stop what you are doing and assume a special pose. All you need to do is to take an internal stance—assume a sense of "coming to" and make an intention to pay attention. If possible, it is helpful to establish a sense of balance, keeping the torso upright, with both feet planted on the ground. No one else need be aware that you are practicing mindfulness.

Sometimes we will want to do a practice somewhere where we won't be disturbed. The "formal" practices on pages 100–139 fall into this category.

There are a few tips on the opposite page that you might like to bear in mind before trying any of the "formal" practices, and they can be applied to many of the other practices throughout the book. If your feet don't easily reach the floor while sitting in a chair, place a cushion or large book underneath then.

If you can't sit in an upright chair or on the floor, simply lie down in any way that feels right for you. Although you may find it harder to stay awake if you are lying down, it is perfectly fine to carry out your practice in this way. Simply lie on the back with arms and legs outstretched and the feet falling away.

Finally, it's a good idea to keep a shawl or blanket nearby that you can wrap around you if you get cold, as our body temperature falls quite quickly when we meditate.

TIPS FOR SITTING UPRIGHT

1   Choose an upright chair rather than an easy chair that does not offer much support. Sit down and, while bending over as if to touch your toes, wriggle your buttocks to the back of the chair, then sit up. This action lifts the spine out of the pelvis without strain. Now imagine an invisible thread that runs from the base of the spine all the way up and along the back of the neck and head and out through the crown of the head. Imagine tugging on this gently, causing your body to lift up slightly and your chin to tuck in.

2   Alternatively, you can sit cross-legged on the floor. It is important to have a stable base, so the hips should be higher than the knees. Ideally, the knees should touch—and so be supported by—the floor. If your knees don't reach the floor, you might want to place some cushions underneath them. If you need to raise your hips, you could place a yoga block, firm cushion, or large book just under the base of the spine to sit on. Then align the spine and head as above..

3   The third option is to kneel, using a meditation stool or cushions. Depending on your height and flexibility, you may need several cushions (if using a stool, you may need to place a yoga block or a few books on top to get some height). We want to avoid a sense of slumping or collapsing as apart from being uncomfortable, our external posture reflects and supports our internal state of mind. When you are in the right position, you will feel perfectly aligned.

4   We are looking for a position of relxed alertness that is grounded (hence both feet remaining on the floor). Place your hands in a comfortable, supported position in your lap—experiment with having your palms up or down. If you keep your eyes open, drop your gaze and rest it slightly in front of you, relaxed rather than staring. When we sit for a period of time we often find that, just as our mind wanders, our pose wanders too. Therefore, checking in with your posture from time to time while sitting down and making any necessary adjustments will support your practice.

CHAPTER TWO

YOU @ WORK

From calming our nerves, encouraging us to see things differently, and noticing the positive experiences, to exploring more helpful and less stressful ways of working, we can discover the transformative power of directing our attention wisely at work.

Mindfulness has the potential to help us in many different types of situations at work. Susan is a solicitor in a busy London firm, a pressurized environment with demanding deadliness. As someone who internalized stress, she came to mindfulness to find a more helpful way to manage challenging times at work.

I was asked to present a sales pitch to a client—this involved going to the client's offices with a presentation and then answering any quick-fire questions they would throw at us to assess whether they wanted to appoint us as their lawyers. I was asked to attend very last minute. I hadn't done many pitches, and aside from the fact that I would be presenting to a potential client, I was also attending the pitch with four partners from our firm. I was one of two junior members of the pitch team and that was almost more terrifying than presenting to the client.

We traveled to the pitch by train and while the others busily buried themselves in their notes, I lowered my eyes, put my palms on my knees, and conducted a breathing space. This instantly calmed me, and I could literally feel my heart rate slow down. I'd worried I would feel self-conscious meditating in front of colleagues, but not one of them noticed—they were all too engrossed in their own preparation. The pitch went very well and the feedback from the client and from my senior colleagues was good. I have no doubt of the part mindfulness played in that.

It is easiest to learn to practice mindfulness when things are going well so that it becomes familiar to us. The more we practice it, the more readily it is available to us when we need it.

IF ONLY...

It is seductive to think that if our circumstances changed all would be well and life would be perfect. However, the more time we spend daydreaming about being somewhere else, the less we pay attention to our job here and now.

Daydreaming creates a sense of dissatisfaction with the present and then we zone out. When we are not present we miss opportunities. These might be chances to interact with colleagues or do something differently. At the most basic level, we are not present for a large part of the working week. Weeks become years and years build into a lifetime. Not being present at work can easily become a habit that we carry home with negative consequences for our family. Paying attention to the present moment with an attitude of curiosity creates an environment of discovery. When we pay attention, we become interested; when we are interested, we discover all kinds of hitherto unknown aspects of our life and the people around us.

TRY THIS

★ Create the intention to notice whenever your thoughts wander off into the fantasy world of "if only."

★ Whenever you become aware that you are daydreaming of the future, bring yourself back to the present by paying attention to your breath (see pages 54 and 78) or the placement of your feet on the floor (see opposite page).

★ It can be helpful to label your thoughts as "daydreaming" at this point of realization.

★ Keep doing this—letting go of any condemnation or judgment about where you have been or the fact that you have been daydreaming.

FEET ON THE FLOOR

This is one of the simplest and most useful practices to do, particularly when things are feeling difficult. The stress reaction (see page 27) can be activated in an instant. A manager tells you off, you realize you've sent an e-mail in error, a customer has been rude to you. Or perhaps something difficult is going on at home—someone you love is sick or a relationship is on the rocks. These are the moments when we feel as if the ground beneath us is falling away and yet, when we are at work, we are expected to be on form and good humored.

One option is to turn our attention to the breath, but when we are panicking our breath becomes shallow and fast. The breath may feel elusive and awareness of this only makes us feel worse. When we feel like this the best thing we can do is to ground ourselves by connecting with the earth beneath us. We can do this most easily through our feet.

Turn your attention to the feet. Do it now. Feel the sensations of your feet in contact with the floor. Push down slightly through the bottom of the feet. It is as if your feet were glued to the floor. The grou solid beneath your feet. Explore these sensations– perhaps a sense of "shoe" or "sock." Wiggle your toes if you'd like to.

When something is weighted at the bottom, it i unlikely to fall over. Focusing your attention to your feet o the floor is like weighting yourself so you don't fall ove You instantly bring yourself into contact with the prese moment. The sense of groundlessness eases off. T thoughts spinning off into the world of "what ifs" sl down. Whatever is going on is still there, but you are ak to face it from a place of stability and strength.

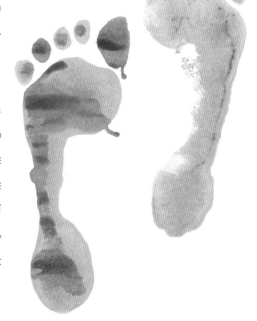

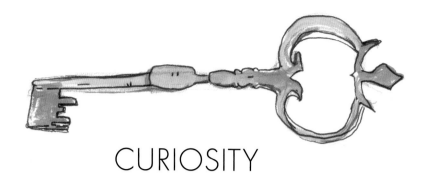

CURIOSITY

Curiosity is a key attitude of mindfulness. To be curious is to be interested, to want to explore, and to find out more, to look at something a bit more closely. In mindfulness, our curiosity should be without expectations of finding out something particular. We want to be curious with beginner's mind—we have no idea what we might find. When we explore something with curious interest, we often discover things we were unaware of—this may be physical sensations, certain emotions or motivations, and we might even notice things about other people.

Children are inherently curious. As we grow older, things we encounter become more familiar and we often take what we experience at face value, ignoring all the layers underneath. If we have been in a particular role at work for a while, or with the same company, we get used to a certain way of doing things. We put up with systems and models that can be clunky because "that's the way we've always done it." When someone new comes along, they tend to be more curious and question the status quo, or perhaps suggest a different way of doing something. Is there any reason we can't bring that kind of curiosity to our existing job now?

To be curious is to be interested, to want to explore

TRY THIS

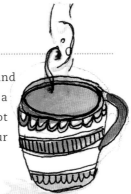

- Today, be curious about *everything*. Assume no foreknowledge and explore your world of work. Ask questions without expecting a particular answer. Talk to people with whom you would not normally converse. Pay attention to the environment, how your colleagues interact with one another and the outside world.

- Be interested in your own experience. Notice what arises, pay attention when there are moments of resistance—a sense of tightness or tension—sometimes this shows up in particular areas of the body. When I get tense at work, I find myself rubbing my neck, which becomes stiff and tight. Where do you hold your tension? Are there particular people or tasks to which your body responds negatively?

- What do you like? Pay attention to those moments when there is a softening, an opening, and a moving towards something. When do you notice this? Are there particular activities, food, beverages, or people that cause this? Is it in response to something that you do?

- Pay attention to specific e-mails, phone calls, and conversations—notice if at any point your body gives you a physical reaction and notice what just happened before. Be interested in any associated thoughts that arose just before, during, or after this reaction. Do you notice any particular emotions? Sometimes there are more than one.

- Pay attention to the feedback that your inner self is giving you via the body. Notice whether there is a contradiction between your thoughts and physical sensations or emotions in your body. Sometimes we find ourselves agreeing to do something or assuring someone we are "fine" and yet at the same time there is a clenching in the gut or a tightening across the shoulders that suggests things are anything but fine.

- Be curious about what you discover about your experience and how you act at work.

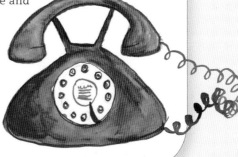

SITTING TALL

My neck and shoulders are the areas that are the first to stiffen. When I pay attention to my posture at work I can see why. My shoulders are scrunched up and my chin is jutting out as I stretch my head towards the computer screen. When I notice how I am sitting, there is an instant softening and letting go. If we can check in with our posture at our desk or in a meeting, we can notice our own habitual patterns. Remember that **it is only when we bring something into awareness that we have the capacity to do it differently.**

TRY THIS

★ Plant your feet flat on the floor. Imagine a silken thread running all the way up the spine, along the back of the neck, and out through the crown of the head. Give this "thread" a gentle tug so that your spine straightens, the crown of the head lifts towards the ceiling, and your chin becomes slightly tucked in. You are now sitting tall, the lower half of the body grounded and connected to the earth beneath your feet and the torso rising up like a mountain peak.

★ Get used to checking in regularly with your posture throughout the day.

★ **Our external posture often reflects our internal state of mind. Notice the connection between the mind and body.**

★ Familiarity with how your posture reflects your state of mind—both positively and negatively—allows you to make adjustments. Consciously **sitting tall can help connect you with the strength of your "inner mountain."**

You can do this practice while standing and walking. Notice how you hold your head and how this influences your mood. Experiment and see what you discover.

WALKING TO WALK

Any activity can become an opportunity for mindfulness practice, particularly moments of transition. Reflect on the amount of times in your day when you have to get from A to B—perhaps to visit a colleague on another floor or collect the post—these "journeys" are often empty moments, but they can become opportunities to do something different. We can turn these periods of "dead time" into practice. When we do this, we move from "doing" into "being" mode, which brings us back into the present moment, creating a mindful pause that can prevent things feeling out of control. This **"bringing ourselves back" then influences how we continue to think and behave.** A small behavioral shift can have a much larger effect. Make the intention to turn these moments of transition into mindfulness practice.

TRY THIS

- As you go from A to B, pay attention to your experience as it unfolds **with interest** and **without judgment**.

- Notice any felt experiences arising—the sensations of your feet on the floor, your hand grasping the door, notice changes in temperature and air, etc.

- Become aware of any thoughts that are present. There might be a sense of anticipation about what is coming next or maybe some nervousness. What does that feel like physically in the body? Where can you feel it? Be curious.

- Acknowledge any emotions that might be present—there may be more than one.

- Be mindful of any encounters with other people. What do you notice?

- You may want to vary your attention, sometimes keeping it tightly focused other times expanding it out to have a wider sense of your environment.

- Do this when you can but recognize that you won't always remember—that's okay.

THOUGHT TONE

I have a particular thought tone that acts as a red flag for me. It is indignant and there is often a sense of self-righteousness about it. When I notice this tone coloring my thoughts, I am aware that my judgment is going to be skewed. I'm taking a fixed stand—and when something is fixed, the viewpoint is always going to be limited. If I can become aware of this thought tone, I can take action, reminding myself that **we all see things differently** and that there may be things going on outside my line of sight.

If you ask half a dozen of witnesses to describe an event you will get six different viewpoints. People are standing in different places, obstacles obstruct the line of sight; people pay attention to what interests them, so one person may notice the label or colors of clothing whereas another is more interested in the music that is playing in the background. When we understand this, we realize that people are not "lying" or deliberately opposing us, but simply acting based on *their* experience, which will be different from yours and mine. This applies to all areas of life. Our personal viewpoint, story line, or opinion is not necessarily the right or the only one. It is just one of various possibilities.

Pay attention to your thought tone. Can you distinguish between different thought tones? Start noticing them—their particular charcteristics. Can you identify those moments when your thinking is overly skewed? There's no need to judge, simply notice it and remind yourself that your judgment may be out of kilter on this occasion. Ground yourself by connecting with the breath (see page 78) or Feet on the Floor (see page 47). Pause. Breathe. Bring yourself back to the present moment—this will act as a brake and give you the opportunity to respond rather than react.

GETTING OUT OF YOUR HEAD

When we are working, most of us spend the majority of time in our head—analyzing, problem-solving, fixing, planning. There is nothing wrong with that when it is suits the task in hand, but too often this becomes our default way of being.

When we get stuck in our head, we are unaware of what's going on in the body and so can miss important early warning signals about our wellbeing. **Being grounded in the body** also **helps prevent us getting swept away by thoughts**. Turning our attention to the body is the quickest way to shift our attention out of the head—away from those repetitive thoughts—and into the body, thereby bringing us into the present moment.

SIMPLE BODY SCAN

1   In your mind's eye, draw an outline around your feet where they are in contact with the floor. First one foot and then the other, tracing around the edge of your shoe or foot.

2   Move your attention up the body, and wherever the body is in contact with the seat, draw around that area—around the thighs and buttocks, perhaps the middle of the back, possibly the back of the head if it is resting on something. Notice the arms—and if they are in contact with anything (even your body) just mentally outline them.

3   Then drop your attention to the feet. Imagine bandaging the feet with a strip of cloth or string. In your mind's eye, wrap your attention around the feet, ankles, lower leg, gradually moving up one leg and then starting again on the opposite side.

4   You can continue as far as you want to—perhaps wrapping the torso and the arms. You can wrap the hands as a whole or wrap individual fingers and thumbs.

This practice is a way of turning your attention to the body. It can be as simple or as complex as you wish. For example, you could just do your feet or hands if you only have a few minutes. Do this as often as you can to bring yourself into the present moment.

THE MINDFUL MINUTE

"I don't have time to practice at work," is a common refrain, but we all have a minute. Michael Chaskalson describes this practice in *The Mindful Workplace*, and it's the perfect antidote to the lack-of-time excuse. People often feel uncomfortable with the open-ended nature of meditation—particularly if they are doing it in the workplace. What I like about this one is that **you can create a simple and time-limited meditation** tailored to you that can be done anywhere. Simply work out the number of breaths you normally take in a minute and use this as a guide to take a Mindful Minute at work.

TRY THIS

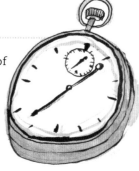

★ You will need a stopwatch or timer to determine the number of breaths taken in a minute. You may want to engage someone else's help with this so you are not worrying about when to start or finish. If you are timing yourself, I'd recommend settling yourself for a moment or two before beginning to watch the clock or timer. When you are ready, begin.

★ Count every breath you take—breathing in and breathing out counts as one breath. Don't worry about the number as we all breathe at different rates. This is to determine the number of breaths you take in a minute, not someone else (and it can vary hugely—in one group of 14 people, for example, it ranged from 7 to 15 breaths).

★ If you like you can always repeat it a couple of times to get an average.

★ Once you have your figure simply remember it and the next time you want to practice, settle your attention on your breath and count each in- and out-breath as one up to the number you determined. That is your Mindful Minute. If you can do this every so often throughout the day, you will be creating minutes of present-moment awareness with all the positive benefits this brings.

OPENING TO THE GOOD

Have you noticed how you are more likely to remember something unpleasant or bad that happens?. We are programmed to be vigilant to any threat—this is what has enabled humans as a species (and each one of us as individuals) to survive. However, too often what we perceive as "threats" are far from it. We might miss our cue in a presentation at work or perhaps it's something we hear a colleague say. Our positive experiences, on the other hand, serve no life-saving function, so the body/mind does not store them in the same way. So we tend to forget anything that is positive and over-emphasize negative experiences. If we can notice a positive experience as it happens we can "bank" it in the body memory. This is not about manufacturing positive experiences but becoming aware of those that are already occurring.

TRY THIS

- For today, notice any experience that you judge as good. We are talking about the small experiences, such as a smile from a friend or a stretch of the body after being hunched over the computer—something that makes you feel good.

- Pay attention to the experience as it is happening. Allow yourself to *feel* it. What physical sensations fo you notice? Are they located in a particular area? How would you describe them? What thoughts are you aware of (no need to judge them)? What emotions? This check-in process need take only seconds.

- It can be helpful to write down your experiences. Reflect on what you noticed—what surprised you? Are there particular tasks or people that you respond to positively?

- Often we realize that actually there are far more pleasant experiences in our day than we thought—even at work. By noticing them we are acknowledging a more balanced view of our life and storing them in the body's emotional memory.

OPENING TO THE DIFFICULT

None of us likes it when life does not go according to plan—we don't like it when the printer jams or the IT department tells us to restart the computer before they'll investigate the error message flashing on the screen. We don't like it when someone repeatedly ignores our phone calls or e-mails, or responds negatively to an idea we have. It is often these small, petty irritations that cause us more stress than the big crises, such as the threat of redundancy or restructure.

Our natural response to anything that we don't like is to resist it—we get irritated or even angry, our body becomes stiff with tension, our blood pressure rises as the heart beats faster in response to a perceived threat (see page 27). We may try and steamroller our way through whatever is going on so we can feel okay as quickly as possible. Although it may seem counter-intuitive, there is much value—both physically and psychologically—to be had from turning our attention to our experience in those moments when things aren't going our way.

Research suggests that we respond to our experience in either "approach" or "avoid" mode. Experiments have shown that when we operate in avoidance mode, we score 50 percent less on creativity tests done immediately afterwards compared to those doing the same activity in approach mode. When we feel threatened (mentally or physically), we activate the stress response (see page 28), which can inhibit the creation of new brain cells (usually occurring every day) as well as neural branching. So avoidance mode has a negative impact on our brain cells, thereby inhibiting the development of new ways of thinking and keeping us stuck in fearful, negative thinking.

ACKNOWLEDGING THE UNWANTED

1 Pay attention to any experience today that you judge as unpleasant, unwanted, or difficult. When you notice that flash of irritation or anger, notice and acknowledge it—**"I see you [name the emotion if you can]."** Don't worry about whether you feel that emotion is inappropriate or not, it is there so accepting its presence through acknowledgment is a crucial first step. Labeling the emotion in this quick way also inhibits the emotion itself.

2 **Explore any felt sensations** around that emotion—can you feel anything physically? Or perhaps there is simply a numbness or absence of feeling? Explore the boundary of any sensation or absence of it. There may be no sensations in the torso, for example, but perhaps you are aware of the feeling of your feet on the floor or buttocks on the chair. Become aware of the story you are telling yourself—let go of any judgments around it.

3 Now **bring your attention to the breath**—perhaps repeating silently to yourself "breathing in / breathing out," or silently saying "it's okay to allow myself to feel this."

4 Stay with the breath for a minute or two and then **gradually expand your awareness**, becoming aware of the body, the feet on the floor, buttocks on the seat, sounds, and other sensations around you before continuing with your day.

If at any time you feel overwhelmed, drop your attention to feeling the feet on the floor. When we say "it's okay," it's important to understand that we are not condoning whatever is going on or saying that it is okay—because it may well not be. What we are doing is acknowledging that this is how we are feeling—it is our experience—and acknowledgment leads to acceptance. The process of tuning into our experience is one of "approach" rather than "avoidance." Turning toward our experience isn't easy if it something we find unpleasant. Practice tuning into any any experience—the good and the neutral, too—as these have less of an emotional charge, and so resistance. Sometimes we are not in a position where we feel safe enough to turn toward a difficult emotion arising. In situations like this it is fine to acknowledge and label how you are feeling, but give yourself permission to come back to it another time (see page 128), for example at home, where you have some time and privacy.

SOUL FOOD

The body needs fuel to operate productively and, just like a car, fuel comes in different grades. If you grab something processed for lunch and snack on donuts, your body's engine will respond in kind. Pay attention to what happens to your mood in the hours after eating. A sugar high might lift you in that moment but you will come crashing down a couple of hours later—and your mood with it. Notice how you feel whenever you skip a meal. How does it affect you, particularly your mood?

When we pay attention to our experience we notice that it often changes. Our senses become more acute, and in eating this affects taste and smell in particular. If what we are eating is flavorsome with interesting textures and smells, slowing down to eat for the sake of eating becomes a rich experience.

There is a time lag between eating and the brain receiving the message that the stomach is full. When we eat too quickly or are distracted, we don't create the opportunity to receive this message. However, when we take our time, we notice when the body says "enough," and because we are aware of the experience, the food seems much more fulfilling than usual. Therefore, when we eat mindfully, we usually eat less because we are listening to the body.

You don't need to find extra time in your day to eat something mindfully

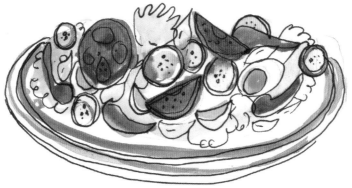

MINDFUL EATING

If you are doing this for the first time, perhaps start with just one item, a piece of fruit for example. Hold it in your hand. Explore it visually—imagine you have never seen something like this before. Notice its color and any surface patterns; become aware of its shape and feel its weight in your hand. Perhaps touch it, feel its texture, then become aware of any smell—hold the object close to the nose. Notice any response in the body to any action. Try holding the object close to the mouth, the lips. What do you notice?

Throughout, pay attention to any thoughts, emotions, or physical sensations in the body. Make a conscious decision to place the item in your mouth and just hold it there —refrain from chewing and simply explore it with your tongue. When you are ready, make an intention to bite into the object. Become aware of any sounds and tastes. Notice when biting becomes chewing—and at some point swallowing. What does that feel like?

Begin to pay attention to your normal mode of eating at work. What do you snack on and when? What do you eat for lunch and where do you eat it? When you are eating, do you simply eat or are you multi-tasking? Pay attention to how you feel immediately after eating and then a couple of hours later. Notice your mood as well as physical sensations in the body and whether you feel alert or sleepy and sluggish. Make an intention to eat your lunch or a snack mindfully. How does that feel? When you snack at work, see if you can bring those moments of choice into awareness. What is driving you to reach for that biscuit or cake? Noticing what precedes an action can be informative—is it boredom or is it in response to something else that has happened? Pausing and noticing your thoughts, emotions, and physical sensations can give you important feedback. You may still eat the biscuit, but it becomes a choice rather than an unconscious, automatic reaction.

GIVE YOURSELF A HUG

Oxytocin is sometimes called the "cuddle hormone" because it increases feelings of optimism, trust, and self-esteem. It activates the calming response, which will turn off the stress reaction and all its unpleasant side effects (see page 27). Hugging a colleague is probably inappropriate, but this practice is something you can do when you are feeling in need of a hug. You could do this practice somewhere quiet and preferably away from people—the bathroom is always a good option.

TRY THIS

★ Begin by settling your attention on the breath. Allow yourself to experience the sensations of breathing and how the body responds.

★ Place one hand on the belly, just below the belly button, and exert gentle pressure. Place the opposite hand over the heart space on the left side of the chest.

★ Keeping the hands in place, focus on the breath. Keep a narrow beam of awareness on the breath, chest, and belly. Really feel the rise and fall and the expansion and contraction.

★ Continue for as long as you wish.

★ The gentle pressure on the heart space and the belly stimulates the release of oxytocin along with its benefits.

Remember—you need to let go of any expectations or desire to make an uncomfortable or unpleasant feeling go away. Mindfulness is about learning to be with whatever arises. Use this practice as a way of connecting with the body and with how you are feeling. Acknowledging that you are in need of a bit of kindness and self-care is an important step.

MULTI-TASKING

Multi-tasking is often applauded. We answer the phone while signing letters or carry on a conversation with a colleague while finishing an e-mail. However, these activities all use the same neural circuits and become overloaded when we try to do too many things at once. Our brain works best when actions are done sequentially.

Performance benefits from focused attention. When we pay attention, we notice things both internally and externally, and we are able to have a greater awareness of what is going on. When we do more than one activity at a time, we are constantly switching our attention between competing tasks. Our attention is split, which causes us to miss things and negatively affects our memory, as every time we come back to one task we have to get our working memory up to speed again. This takes time and is mentally exhausting because our brain has to work a lot harder to get the same results. This uses up energy, so our productivity declines a lot more quickly and we are more likely to make mistakes as our memory is impaired.

TRY THIS

- Notice how you feel when you multi-task, how it affects your work in the moment.

- Become aware of when you are multi-tasking and, if possible, pause, gently reminding yourself that you are trying to do something different.

- Multi-tasking is a habit, so it will take a bit of time to change. Don't be too hard on yourself when you forget—rather, celebrate the times when you remember.

- If you have to multi-task, mix the tasks wisely. Combine a task that uses the pre-frontal cortex—the thinking brain—with one that is more routine-oriented. Routine-oriented tasks are "learned" and have become automatic and embedded in the basal ganglia of the brain. We can do these tasks without thinking, so they take up less energy.

THE POWER OF CHOICE

One of the characteristics of stress is feeling powerless. At work, we can often feel like a cog in a machine—our start and end times are determined, and sometimes even when we can take a break or go to the toilet is regulated by the "powers that be." Introducing choice can be helpful when we have a choice about something, it feels more manageable because we are in approach mode rather than the avoidance mode that inhibits creative thinking and keeps us stuck in a fearful mode of mind. When we are resisting something, we activate our "threat" mode with all that this entails (see page 25). We can activate the limbic system—the part of the brain that regulates emotion and memory and includes the amygdala—in a positive way by finding a way to make a choice in a stressful situation.

EXPLORING CHOICES

★ Look for any choice, however small, such as choosing the time for a meeting.

★ If you are being forced to go down a particular route at work, look for something positive that you are getting out of the situation. How will this particular decision benefit you? There may be a financial payoff, or an opportunity to spend more time at home. Can you look at the situation with fresh eyes and see it differently?

★ You have the power to choose how you respond to any situation. You can choose to be a victim or you can take responsibility for your own state of mind. Notice the stories you are telling yourself—how are you describing it? What role do you cast yourself in? If you feel stuck in your thoughts, shift your attention to the body, the breath, the feet on the floor, and every time the story pulls you away just bring your attention back to the point of focus. Make a deliberate choice about where you place your attention.

WORKING WITH HABITS

Habits are a learned set of behaviors. They are routine and we do them without awareness. For a set of behaviors to become a habit, the brain shifts control from the top of the head to the bottom, the basal ganglia. This area automatically controls routine activities, without conscious awareness. To reverse a habit, we have to bring it back into our consciousness, become aware of its particular triggers and choose to do something different. We need self-awareness, and this is cultivated through mindfulness practice by regularly bringing our attention to our experience as it unfolds.

TRY THIS

Decide on something that has become a habit that you would like to change. It could be checking your e-mails every few minutes, for example.

- When you do become aware of the impulse to act in the habitual way—notice it. Where do you feel it in the body? What are you thinking of? What is driving the behavior? Notice any emotions such as boredom, restlessness, or fear.

- Remind yourself that you have a choice about what to do next. What alternatives are available to you and what is the wisest option for you to take in the moment?

- Remember that to begin with, our awareness often kicks in after or during the event rather than before. This is perfectly normal. Be gentle with yourself and, if it's possible, stop the unhelpful habit in the very moment you realize you are doing it.

The more we can do something differently, the better able we are to establish newly embedded patterns of behavior. The more you practice checking in with yourself and bringing yourself into the present moment, for example, the more these practices become embedded into the basal ganglia. You will find yourself doing them without consciously initiating them. We do, however want to let go of any automatic behaviours that are not particularly helpful.

WORKING OUT THE SENSES

When we pay attention to what is happening, we are opening up to our whole experience in as wide a way as possible. To help us do this, we want to get used to tuning in to all our five senses—taste, touch, sound, sight, and smell. We are used to activating some of these more than others, so if we can make a conscious effort to use all five senses, we begin to stimulate all of them—including those that are underused.

The Narrative Path

In his book *Your Brain at Work*, David Rock explains how we usually operate either along a narrative path (dominated by thoughts and the story we are telling ourselves about our experience) or along one of direct-experience (paying attention to our experience through the senses). For most people, the narrative path is the default.

We think about our experience and that thought leads to another and then another, rather than actually being aware of the experience in that very moment. However, if we can activate the direct-experience network, we begin to perceive so much more. More information becomes available to us through our senses, and this creates more options and choices, which make us more effective.

People who meditate regularly find it easier to notice when they are stuck on the narrative path—operating within past habits and expectations, for example, and they can deliberately turn their attention to their present-moment experience. But we do have to practice tuning in to our experience, and this little practice is one to do regularly. It's a great one to do in different environments—outside, in a meeting room, on the shop floor, in a café—select locations that will stimulate different senses.

TRY THIS

★ As you become aware of an experience—it could be drinking a cup of coffee at your desk, for example, or perhaps taking a walk at lunchtime—make a deliberate intention to engage all your senses. Begin with any one of them, usually the most dominant one. For example, if you are drinking a cup of coffee, notice the warmth of the cup in your hands (**touch**). Then become aware of the aroma of the fresh coffee (**smell**) and the flavor of the coffee in your mouth (**taste**)—both in the moment the liquid enters the mouth and hits the taste buds and you're tasting it as well as the after taste, notice the difference between these. They are three obvious senses we engage—but what about the **sound** of drinking coffee? What do you notice about that? How about the color or tone of your coffee? What do you **see** as you look at it?

★ You can begin by focusing tightly on your cup of coffee, then gradually widen your beam of awareness to explore the environment around you with all your five senses.

★ Some senses will always be easier to engage with than others, which may need to be teased and coaxed into awareness. If you really can't identify something, just notice the absence of it. Become aware of any story playing in your head about "not doing it right," "I can't do this," or any other judgmental thoughts. Acknowledge them and notice that you are caught on the "narrative path" and bring your attention back to your direct experience.

★ Bring an attitude of playfulness to this one, and if you find it difficult at first, trust that it will become easier with practice.

BEING IN THE ZONE

When we are performing our best, we are in command of our actions and it feels as if everything is unfolding without any effort. Time seems to stand still and we feel energized and totally absorbed; we are unlikely to be distracted by external or internal "noise." This is sometimes called being in the zone or the flow state, the latter a term coined by Mihaly Csikszentmihalyi in his book *Flow: The Psychology of Optimal Experience*.

Psychologist Martin Seligman suggests that the flow state is one of the three main drivers of human happiness. When we are in flow, our skill set is matched to the task in hand, and because we are good at something, the skills needed for this action have become embedded in the routine-oriented area of our brain (the basal ganglia), so they require minimal effort. Flow is the sweet spot between over-arousal of the pre-frontal cortex and under-arousal (boredom)—the point where we are thriving from the challenge we are facing (see page 25).

Goleman suggests in his book *Focus: the Hidden Driver of Excellence*, that if we deliberately focus our attention on a task, we are more likely to become absorbed in it and move into the flow state. This suggests that our ability to direct our attention intentionally and ignore distractions can enhance our performance. Rather than waiting for the mood to strike us, **we can direct our attention in a particular way**, and the flow state will arise out of this.

Let Go of Distractions

When we practice mindfulness, we are learning how to place our attention in a deliberate way and practicing letting go of distractions (internal and external), thereby improving our ability to concentrate. The more we do it, the more practiced we become, and this is borne out by research.

Neuroscientist Sara Lazar and colleagues showed that people who practice meditation for 40 minutes a day developed a thicker cortex in the areas of the right pre-frontal cortex and the right anterior insula. These are the areas associated with decision-making, attention, and awareness. Furthermore, there was a correlation between the meditation experience of the subjects and the degree of increase.

Increase your ability to move into the flow state by regularly practicing mindfulness. You can do this in the moment as well by establishing a regular practice outside of work hours.

- Do a Mindful Minute (see page 54) if you are at work.

- Exercise your attention muscles by regularly practicing meditations such as Watching the Breath (see page 102).

- A practice such as Watching the Breath and the Body (see page 106) will help cultivate the ability to let go of physical distractions, and Sound versus Noise (see page 126) will aid the ability to shut out external distractions such as noise.

It is also important to choose what **not** to focus on. Internal and external distractions will always be clamoring for attention, which can pull us out of the zone. Here is an opportunity to use the skills learned through mindfulness practice of repeatedly letting go and returning to your point of focus. It is helpful to remember that **this continual letting go and returning to a point of focus is the practice**.

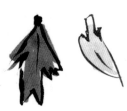
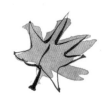

ZONING OUT

If we are unhappy, bored, or unmotivated at work, we are disengaged. Our attention is elsewhere—what we are going to do as soon as we get out that door, our plans for the weekend, the next holiday, the dream job that we will land some day—anything is better than actually being at work. The problem with this is that the underlying feeling of dissatisfaction is very unsettling and will come out in our performance, our interactions with colleagues and customers, and with our family and friends. **We can't always leave our job but we can change the way we perceive it.**

In traditional Buddhist retreats, everyone supports the smooth running of the retreat by offering "work practice"—this might be cleaning the toilets, cooking, doing the dishes, gardening, or any other tasks that need doing. Although there may be an initial reluctance to take on the role of cleaning the toilets, for example, the experience can be transformative as you realize that it is the attitude you bring to the task, rather than the job itself, that is fundamental.

When we **pay attention** to something and **become curious and interested** in it, we begin to see all kinds of things we usually miss. This draws us in further and so we discover more and more.

We discover that our attention has the power to transform our experience, making it feel much richer

TRY THIS

· ·

- Make the workplace and your attitude towards it an opportunity to practice mindfulness. Cast your mind back to when you first got your job. How did you feel? Can you connect with that sense of something new unfolding? Can you take off the scratched filters of your attitude to see your workplace with fresh eyes? Imagine you are a new starter today. How would that feel? What would you be excited about?

- Remind yourself that you have a choice about how you respond to your work.

- Notice when you zone out from work—and make an intention to bring yourself back (time and time again). Identify your top five distractions—eating, chatting, the Internet, your phone, text messaging. Whatever they are, list them and pay attention to the impulse to engage in any one of them. When you become aware of the impulse as a felt sensation in the body, perhaps a sense of an emotion such as boredom or a thought tempting you away, acknowledge its presence and take your attention to the breath. Use it as an anchor to ride out the impulse as best as you can. Even if you can inhibit it for a short while you are gradually re-wiring your brain, so don't give up.

- Remind yourself that you are here anyway, so why not make the best of it. This does not mean gritting your teeth to get through it, but rather bringing a different attitude to your day. **See what happens when you really begin to engage with your work** rather than zone out of it. What do you notice?

- Remind yourself that if you are in a negative frame of mind about work that will skew all your perceptions about it. Open your eyes to all of it—the good, the bad, the boring.

- Focus on the task in hand (even when you don't want to). Notice what effect that has.

- Treat this practice as an experiment—choose a start and end date, ideally long enough so you start seeing a difference. Make the intention and follow it through. When your intentions falter, start again. Try not to judge the experience as you are doing it. At the end of the month, take some time to reflect on how you feel about your job.

GETTING TO KNOW YOUR BRAIN

We are all familiar with the concept that if we over-exercise, we will get physically exhausted. Most of us would avoid planning a day packed full of physical activities as we know our body's limitations. However, we don't usually think about our brains in the same way. Yet the pre-frontal cortex—the area of the brain that deals with decision-making and other higher-level functions—uses up a lot of energy compared to more routine activities such as those done on autopilot.

When the brain's resources are depleted, it will resort to more automatic ways of thinking as this takes up less energy. When we are on autopilot, we are more likely to fall into habitual patterns of thinking and behavior, and these are often unhelpful. Old ways of thinking are also not going to give us the new strategy we need to bring the latest product to market or whatever project it is that we are working on.

If we accept the idea that our higher brain functions are a limited resource, we can begin to think about how best to use them. In *Your Brain at Work*, David Rock emphasizes the importance of this. In order to conserve the brain's resources Rock recommends:

- Scheduling activities according to the degree of attention they require. Therefore, the start of each working day should be spent "prioritizing the prioritizing" as this involves a large amount of decision-making.

- Holding multiple tasks in one's head at any one time is exhausting—two to three is our ideal limit, but the fewer the better. Therefore, writing down your to do list for comparison will use up less energy.

- Think about the different activities you do throughout your day (dealing with e-mails, phone calls, meetings, managing others, talking to customers.)

Schedule those which require a greater degree of concentration or decision-making for when you feel fresh. Bear in mind that if you are working on something new or creative, it will require more brainpower than something that is more routine–oriented.

- Grouping like-minded activities together will make better use of your brain's resources than repeatedly switching back and forth between different types of activity, which becomes distracting.

- Remember to factor in some downtime to allow your brain to rest and reboot. Downtime might be a routine task, such as tidying your desk.

Notice how your attention ebbs and flows through the working day. Make a brief note of different activities, the time of day, the degree and length of time you felt focused, and any other observations. Do this for a week, so you can determine any pattterns in terms of your attention (or lack of it) versus performance.

Begin to implement some of the above strategies, using the information you have gathered about your brain and your average working day. Bring the same attitude of curiosity and experimentation to this stage—what do you notice about working to make best use of your brainpower.

"Your ability to make great decisions is a limited resource. Conserve this resource at every opportunity."

David Rock, *Your Brain at Work*

LABELING

When we do sitting practice, one of the first things we notice is how busy our mind is and how our attention is continually being pulled away by thoughts, emotions, and physical sensations. We are totally swept up in our experience. An image that is sometimes used is that of being in a plane flying through the sky—our emotions are all around us like the clouds and we can't see clearly because we are blinded by the fog around us.

When we don't like what we are experiencing, we often try and suppress it. This takes up a lot of the brain's resources, which means they are diverted from the actual work they are supposed to be doing. We may find that our memory, for example, is affected. When our brain's resources are taxed, it powers down to the easiest mode of processing. This mode is the most automatic of the brain's operating systems and therefore we are more likely to move into a reactive rather than a response mode, with all the behavioral dangers this entails.

Being with Emotions and Thoughts

One of the ways we can practice being with distractions like our thoughts is by labeling them—perhaps as "thinking" or "planning" or "rumination" or "worry." Generally, the recommendation is to keep the description quite broad, otherwise we can get too caught up in trying to find the perfect description of how we are feeling.

It's also helpful to label any emotions we notice—"worry is here," for example. Labeling creates a sense of distance from whatever is going on. We become like a plane, flying above the clouds. The clouds (emotions) are still there but there is a distance between us. Through this witnessing stance we are one step removed from our thoughts or emotions, and we are more likely to see them as passing events rather than identify with them.

🖎 Next time you notice yourself caught up in a particular problem or emotion, try labeling it. For example, "stressed," or "anxious." Remember to use the Feet on the Floor practice (page 47) to connect yourself with the present moment if you need to..

🖎 This practice is not an instant fix. People often think that labeling the emotion will make it disappear like magic. Unfortunately it doesn't work like that. As with all mindfulness practices, this is about learning to be with difficult emotions in a different way rather than getting rid of them completely (which may happen but equally may not), so we want to let go of any expectations of achieving a particular outcome.

Research has shown that when we label our emotions, we activate an area of the pre-frontal cortex that inhibits the automatic response generated by the amygdala (which is associated with negative thinking and emotional reactivity). Therefore **labeling helps prevent negativity from arising**.

There is a distinction between labeling what we are feeling and thinking about it. Labeling is short and symbolic. We do not want to get into a dialogue about how we are feeling, as that runs the risk of turning into rumination. Labeling allows us to be with our emotions because we are using the breath as an anchor at the same time as we observe our thoughts or emotions arising. Thus we see that the particular emotion or thought is just one part of our experience in the same way the breath is.

Once an emotion takes hold it is harder to be with it, so the more you can practice becoming aware of emotions arising, the easier it will be to nip them in the bud. You can do this by becoming familiar with your own body. Regularly tune into the body when you are feeling different emotions. Experiment and do it when you are feeling happy, excited, sad, angry, or frustrated.

MOOD AFFECTS INTERPRETATION

Imagine the following scenario:

Susan had an argument with her partner the night before because despite the risk of redundancy at work he suggested booking a vacation that Susan doesn't think they can afford. This morning there was still tension between them. Now Susan feels bad that they parted without making up.

Susan has just seen Peter, a colleague, come out of the boss's office looking pleased. Then her boss calls her into his office and gives her some feedback on one of her projects. Susan's boss tells her that she did a good job considering it was a first attempt, and suggests some ways for improvement for the next time. When Peter asks Susan how it went, she replies that the boss wasn't pleased. Susan asks Peter about his project and he replies that the boss was really pleased and they had discussed ways it could be even better next time.

Susan knows the business is under pressure and wonders if their boss has been asked to make departmental cuts. Maybe the task they had been given was actually a test and she messed it up. Susan thinks about what would happen if both she and her partner lost their jobs. No vacation this year—and what about the mortgage? Suddenly a lifetime of missed mortgage payments and overdue credit card bills rears up in front of her. She imagines the house being re-possessed, her relationship breaking down and, as a single mum, landing on her mother's front-door step with a suitcase, two kids, the dog, and a goldfish in tow...

This kind of catastrophizing is very common. The mood we are in will affect how we interpret an event and thus the story we tell ourselves. Susan was feeling down because of the argument with her partner, along with a nagging anxiety about his possible redundancy. She went into the meeting with her boss feeling anxious and so she focused on the negative things and ignored any positive feedback. Not only does our mood influence our interpretation of

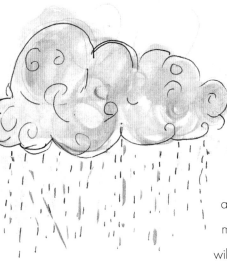

events, but our brain also discounts information that does not corroborate the particular interpretation for which we are looking. If we are feeling stressed we will only pay attention to facts that support our version of the story.

Through regularly practicing mindfulness we become aware of the habitual thought stories that we tell ourselves. The more we can pay attention to our experience, the more likely we will be able to identify our mood and notice the many opportunities where we can apply our mindfulness practice.

For example, what are the top ten tunes you constantly play in your head? The more we see the repetitive nature of these thoughts, the more we can see them just as stories, and eventually we get bored. Know that your mood is going to affect your interpretation and take account of this bias. Acknowledge your mood, particularly if it is low, test your interpretation, and consider what other options there might be.

Notice how quickly a negative thought can spiral out of control and, at the first sense of this happening, STOP. Drop your attention to your breath or the feet on the floor. Pay attention to the breath and every time you notice your thoughts pulling you away, just come right back.

If your mood is down, **acknowledge how you are feeling**. What could you do to look after yourself? Sometimes a change of perspective as simple as looking out of a window can help. Having a chat with a friend is an opportunity to get another opinion, but be aware of how you are recounting the story. What are you emphasizing? Can you present it in a neutral way?

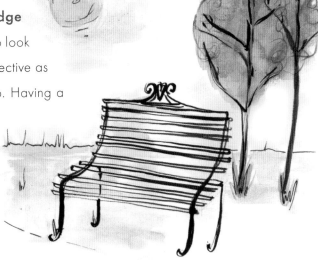

THE TYRANNY OF PERFECTIONISM

We are often our hardest taskmaster—demanding more and expecting higher standards than we would ever dream of asking of a colleague. The bad news for the perfectionist is that you are never going to get there—you will always feel as if you could have done better or worked harder.

This constant judging of oneself and falling short of expectations is exhausting and undermines one's confidence and self-esteem. Often we want everything to be perfect as a way of keeping control, but life, and particularly life at work, is always beyond our control. As we feel control slipping away, we work harder and demand more of ourselves in an attempt to keep hold, but it is like running on a treadmill that someone has turned up to full speed—we can run faster to keep up at first, but at some point we will trip up.

TRY THIS

Begin to pay attention to those moments when you feel pressured. Perhaps it is about delivering a particular project or maybe it is a constant feeling when you are at work.

★ What thoughts are on your mind?

★ What stories are you telling yourself about this task and your role in it?

★ What emotions are present?

★ What physical sensations are arising?

Be curious about when you notice this behavior arising. What do you discover? Is it linked to particular tasks or periods at work? How do you behave toward others when you are feeling this way? How do you behave toward yourself—do you ease off or press the accelerator to achieve more? How does it affect you outside work—your sleeping and eating patterns and your social activities? How often do episodes like that happen at work? Perhaps keep a note for a week to see what patterns may arise.

Once we deliberately begin to bring a particular behavior into our awareness, we are in a much stronger position to do something about it. So if we can become familiar with this pressured quality and how it feels (see practice on the opposite page), we are more likely to notice it as it begins to emerge.

This is the point to take action: to pause and notice it—turning your attention to what you are experiencing. Notice in particular the thoughts—and what is driving you—and perhaps challenge or reframe them. Use the Breathing Space (see page 78) to bring yourself out of the automatic doing mode and into being mode where you can take wise action.

One of the benefits of doing practices such as Watching the Breath (see page 102), Watching the Breath and Body (see page 106), or Sitting with Upset (see page 128), is that we are learning to be more comfortable with change. We are learning to **let go of needing to control our experience** and, instead, be with whatever arises—even the bits we don't like, as we realize that focusing on the breath and body is an anchor that keeps us from getting swept away.

This is how the skills we learn in formal sitting practice can be transferred to our workplace. We remind ourselves that we have done this before. We remind ourselves that **our thoughts are not facts and we don't have to take them as truth**. Through sitting we practice bringing back the wandering mind without condemnation and criticism. Letting go of that constant self-judging is as important as bringing the attention back.

It is also helpful to remind ourselves that this is good enough. Not in the sense of settling for a poor-quality job, but acknowledging that it is only possible to do so much with the particular personal resources we have. The workplace is all about allocating resources appropriately and this applies to your own resources, too. Use—and conserve—your resources wisely and they will go further.

CREATING SPACE WITH THE BREATH

The Breathing Space is a mini meditation that is particularly useful in the workplace. It can be done any time and anywhere and no one need be aware that you are doing it. It is easiest to see it as a three-step process. This is a practice to bring you into the present moment—to shift out of "doing" mode into "being" mode, rather than making whatever we are feeling go away.

Step 1: Check in with how you are and acknowledge what you find there. Notice your thoughts, any emotions that are present, and any physical sensations in the body (Head/Heart/Body). This honest acknowledgment is crucial and must not be ignored. You may not like the thoughts or feelings that are arising or you might feel they are inappropriate, but the reality is that this is what you are feeling. We can only move forward when we know from where we are starting.

Step 2: Bring your attention to the breath wherever you feel it most strongly—this might be the belly or chest, or possibly around the nostrils or upper lip. Stay with the length of each in-breath, noticing the pause when an in-breath becomes an out-breath, and then pay attention to the out-breath. Sometimes it can be helpful to repeat silently to yourself "breathing in... breathing out."

Step 3: Begin to expand your awareness from focusing solely on the breath, and include the body, your feet on the floor, perhaps sounds in the room, smells. Expand your attention wider and wider.

The breath gives us some space. I often think of our thoughts and feelings as a tangled skein of knitting yarn, all knotted up so the individual pieces and colors are indistinguishable and it's one hard solid mass. The breath begins the process of loosening the knots and letting in some space, light, and air. The skein may still be tangled but it's more open and spacious and we can begin to see individual yarns, their colors, and textures.

Just as when we pay attention to our experience—rather than just seeing "anger" or "sadness" we begin to see individual elements, a sick feeling in the stomach, tension around the neck, a racing heart, clenched fists or jaw—we notice particular thoughts. "I'm going to lose my job" or "We've lost that order because I made that mistake." We may notice anger, for example, but possibly also fear or other emotions. Noticing our unfolding experience in such a manner is like unpacking a suitcase. All the elements are still there but we can see them more clearly for what they are.

The Breathing Space is a good practice to do as often as possible, however, the most difficult thing is remembering to do it. It's helpful to tack it on to some activity that you are already doing, such as a mealtime, going up in the elevator, or taking a coffee break. It does not matter what it is, but choose something you do regularly. You might still forget to do it, but the fact that you did schedule it means that at some point you will remember that you have forgotten to do it—that moment is the time to do a Breathing Space! The more you do it, the more often it will occur to you to do it.

In Times of Trouble

We can do a Breathing Space in times of trouble when we are feeling stressed or panicky. As we are focusing on the breath, we can repeat silently to ourselves—"It's okay. I'm okay." When we do this "self-soothing," it is a bit like holding a crying child. We are not saying that whatever the situation that has made us upset is okay, but we are acknowledging that it is okay for us to be sad, upset, afraid, or whatever emotions we might be experiencing. We are holding our feelings with kindness and compassion as we breathe alongside them.

We can also do a Breathing Space and then ask, "what would be the wise thing for me to do now?" This might be removing yourself from the situation. It might be doing something that feels nourishing to make yourself feel better. You might decide to get some support through talking to a friend or colleague. You may decide to do nothing until you have a better idea of what the right thing to do might be. Whatever it is, it is the result of you deliberately asking yourself "what do I need to do to take care of myself right now?"

CHAPTER THREE

YOU AND OTHERS @ WORK

Work is about relationships: relationships with colleagues, customers, clients, service providers, and suppliers underpin everything and can be the difference between a job being well done or not—and how both parties feel about it. The more we can bring awareness to these relationships and to how we interact within them, the better it is for everyone.

Kate came to mindfulness because she found herself getting wound up by colleagues. As she started using mindfulness at work, she became aware of a specific person who pushed her buttons, and she noticed how the irritation would stay with her long after the interaction with that person was over. Describing one encounter with the individual, she said:

> "When I started practicing mindfulness I never used to notice any physical sensations in my body, but more recently I've become aware of my irritation as it arises because I become very hot all over. As well as noticing this as it happens, I am now able to take a step back and actually steer the discussion. In a recent meeting with this person, I found that I was noticing good things about her, such as her nice features and expression, whereas previously I had just seen her as a 'difficult person.' Now I can see more than that—I can see what is good about her. Since I've been practicing mindfulness over the last few weeks, I've noticed that I have a sense of kindness and compassion as well as having become aware of my own particular pressure points."

The qualities of kindness and compassion arose out of Kate's practice. Regularly tuning into the body during meditation practice meant she was attuned to any physical changes arising and this feedback proved invaluable as it allowed her to take control. Kate's practice changed her behavior and that in turn changes how individuals will respond. It's important to be patient with mindfulness, however, we start to see results if we practice regularly, which encourages us to keep going.

BEING IN CONVERSATION

When we are in conversation, we are often working to our own agenda—not necessarily in an intentionally manipulative way, but often because we have our sight set on a particular outcome. This can lead to tunnel vision and a reluctance to be open to other possibilities that might arise. When this occurs, both parties can leave the conversation feeling as if none of their needs has been met. However, there is a different way. What if we really paid attention and listened to what was being said and responded from that moment?

We often make assumptions about what the other person is going to say, and we rehearse our response either before or while the other person is speaking. This means that often we are not even paying attention to what is actually being said. When both parties do this, there is no meaningful dialogue and the conversation can quickly turn into a competition to see who can get their point across loudest.

When we make the intention to listen deeply, we listen with all of our senses. Consequently, we hear much more because we are paying attention to the speaker's body language as well as his or her words. **If we regularly check in with our body and notice what we are feeling physically and emotionally, we are much more likely to respond from the present moment to what was actually said rather than react automatically to what we think we heard or what we expected to hear.** We are also more likely to respond from a place of authenticity as we are in touch with our own feelings about the topic. When we feel heard, we are much more likely to feel positive about the exchange, even if the outcome does not go our way.

TRY THIS

★ Think about your underlying intention for the conversation. What is it?

★ Take a moment to ground yourself by paying attention to your feet on the floor, your buttocks on the seat, and lightly rest your attention on the breath. **Checking in regularly with your felt experience will anchor you in the present moment.**

★ When the other person is speaking, really listen. Pay attention to their words and body language. The two may not always match up.

★ Pay attention to your own experience throughout, and particularly while listening. What thoughts, emotions, and physical sensations in the body are you recognizing? Notice in particular what you react to and whether there is any sense of "not wanting," of unease or resistance. **Keep touching base with your body anchor.**

★ Notice whether there is an urge to interrupt or "tell your story," and resist by staying in touch with the breath and body.

★ When the speaker has finished, pause and take a moment to check in with yourself before responding.

★ Bearing in mind your over-arching intention, respond to what the other person *actually* said—rather than what you thought they were going to say.

★ Remember that it is okay not to say anything and to allow silence.

★ Carry on in this manner. Listen deeply, pay attention to your own experience, and regularly check in with your body anchor.

★ **Be kind to yourself when you forget and interrupt.**

★ Repeat the last two steps over and over again!

Mindful listening is not easy and can be hijacked easily by your emotions, so be patient and see this as an ongoing practice. You may notice that the mood you are in can also affect how easily you are able to practice this. Bear this in mind if you have to have a difficult conversation. At first, you may only be able to listen mindfully for short periods of time, but with practice and intention it will get easier.

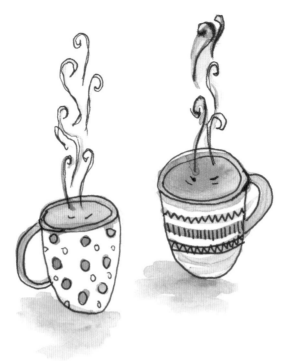

LISTENING DEEPLY

Listening deeply is a difficult skill, particularly when someone is sharing something painful. In some jobs, such as the caring professions or support services, being there for people who are suffering is a daily occurrence and requires particular training.

Regardless of your work, many of us may still come into contact with people who are upset, and we may feel unsure about how to help them. Hearing of someone else's suffering may make us feel uncomfortable. It may stir up feelings in ourselves that we don't like. We may feel awkward and worry about the right thing to say or do, and be afraid of making things worse. We may offer solutions to fix the problem. However, many problems can't be fixed and often the speaker simply wants the opportunity to be heard We can be a witness by using mindfulness to be there for them, but without taking on their suffering so it becomes ours. Being with someone else's pain requires presence and the ability to stay grounded. You can cultivate this by doing a regular sitting practice, however short (see pages 102–109).

TRY THIS

- Use your body as an anchor to bring you into the present moment.

- Listen to what is being said—*really* listen. Notice any response that arises in your own body. Use the breath to keep you grounded.

- Take your cue from the other person about how much he or she wants to share or even just talk. Avoid exerting any pressure to do so.

- Offer the other person space and choice—does she want you to be there with her? Would he prefer to be on his own or perhaps with a friend?

- Notice whether there is an urge to jump in and "fix it." Use your breath and body to resist and instead reflect upon, as best as you can, what is being said to you (for example: "It sounds as if you are...").

- Avoid interrupting by saying "I know how you feel..." or by topping the story with something worse that happened to you.

- If you are not sure what to say—acknowledge that, but don't put the burden on the other person to make you feel better.

- Tune into your own felt experience, notice any thoughts, emotions, and sensations, and breathe with them. Connect with your feet on the floor.

- If emotions such as frustration and impatience are arising, silently acknowledge them while paying attention to the breath.

- You can deliberately breathe in their pain and suffering, and on your out-breath, breathe out peace, calm, or any words you think would be helpful. This can help give us a sense of purpose in a situation in which we often feel helpless.

- When you are on your own, take a few moments to check in with yourself making sure you do whatever is needed to take care of yourself.

THE DIFFICULT PERSON

There will always be people at work who push our buttons. Sometimes we know why but often we don't—they just annoy us and we react negatively to them. This can have consequences for us personally as well as professionally. When we have a negative encounter with someone who winds us up, it doesn't make us feel good about ourselves. We can revisit the experience countless times in our head—and every time we do, we re-live that experience, both physically and emotionally, as if it were actually happening.

If the person is a member of our team, a client or customer, or someone we come into regular contact with, an uncomfortable relationship can cause friction and dissonance that ripples out. Perhaps you won't get that contract or order; perhaps a talented colleague will move on rather than work in such an environment. You might be labeled as "not a team player."

Is there someone you can identify in your work who is causing you problems? If so, the place to start is not with them but with you.

Remember that when we are on autopilot, we are more likely to react to having our buttons pressed, so the more we can do to bring ourselves into the present moment, the less likely this going to happen. We can do this in a general way by practicing mindfulness as much as we can, following any of the practices in this book. However, you can also intentionally do it before or during any interactions with this person.

Practices you can do easily before a meeting, phone call, or e-mail include a Mindful Minute (see page 54). Another practice you could do during an encounter, without the other person even being aware of it, is Feet on the Floor (see page 47). These practices will ground you in the present moment and thus shift you out of "doing" mode (where you are more likely to react) and into "being" mode (where you are more likely to respond).

Opportunity vs. Obstacle

It can be helpful to view the other person as an opportunity for practice rather than an obstacle or inconvenience. Be curious—notice how you feel physically in any encounter with them. Notice differences between live interactions versus e-mail or phone conversations. What thoughts do you notice—what story are you telling yourself about this person? What evidence is there to support your story? How does the mood you are in affect how you are feeling? View your interactions as an experiment—notice your mood before and after, and how your mood affects them.

What can you do differently? How is your body language? Often we behave differently with someone we find difficult—there is a resistance in us to which the other person reacts. Perhaps we don't indulge in the "how was your weekend" type of conversation that we do with other colleagues—these types of interaction enable us to see colleagues as individuals with their own lives. You might discover a common interest or realize there is something difficult going on in their life, such as sick relative or a home renovation, which is making them stressed.

Be mindful of your ego and whether it's getting in the way. We all have a sense of identity and this is often particularly strong at work where we are defined by our job title, for example. We may have a particular view of ourselves in the work hierarchy that we want to protect, or we may feel undervalued—but is that really true? What if we can let that go? Be alert to your ego and when you notice it rearing its head and shouting "Me! Me!" pause, pay attention, and practice letting it go.

Good relationships are crucial at work but it can be helpful to remember that we don't have to like someone to have a good working relationship with them.

THE POWER OF INTENTION

When we make a considered decision to act in a particular way, we are instantly moving out of autopilot and into the present moment. We are saying that **we want to choose how we respond.** This does not mean that we won't get hijacked by an emotional response along the way, but the chances of this occurring are lessened if we can start out and maintain a clear sense of what our intention is.

When we "sit" in meditation practice, we begin by making a clear intention to ourselves about where we are going to place our attention. It might be on the breath, the body, sounds we hear, or our thoughts, or opening up to whatever comes into our awareness. If we choose the breath, we then might drill down further and decide to focus our attention on a particular location. Thus something we do in formal practice—setting an intention and then deliberately working with that intention—can be transferred to everyday life.

Awareness of Attitude

When we interact with other people at work, we often come to the exchange with a particular attitude. We may have specific expectations about what we want from them, a distinct agenda, a personal territory or role to protect—literally or metaphorically—and our ego often gets in the way. If our intention is negative, this is going to influence everything that follows, whereas if we can use intention to guide our way, the outcome may be very different.

For example, a senior manager might have to make the difficult decision to lay off a member of staff due to the economic climate. It's an unpleasant task but if the manager can go into the process with the over-riding intention to treat the member of staff with respect and kindness, that will be felt by the staff member on the receiving end.

Sometimes we can go into a meeting with the intention of behaving in a particular way but find that our behavior gets hijacked by our emotions. If you become aware of this, bring your attention to the Feet on the Floor (see page 47) or the breath to bring yourself into the present moment, and remind yourself of the intention you made before the meeting. Pause and move forward from that place of intention once more. You may have to do this several times as it is not easy.

- Explore what your intention is when you interact with others face to face or through e-mails or on the phone. Is your intention to hurt, wound, score a point, vent some anger? If those emotions are driving your thoughts and actions, perhaps they are clouding your judgment and it might be more appropriate to wait until you are feeling in a more balanced frame of mind. We are always interested in just noticing what is there rather than judging it, so if you do become aware of a negative intention, refrain from beating yourself up about it. Acknowledge it and move on without adding a narrative to it.

- You can make a particular intention at the start of the day, for example, to act with kindness towards others or to open to the good that is in your life—you can choose anything you would like to explore. It can be helpful to write it down as the act of writing something down helps strengthen the intention.

- At the end of the day reflect on what you noticed. In her book *Taking the Leap*, Pema Chodron describes Dzigar Kongrul Rinpoche's teachings: *"When he sees that he has connected with his aspiration even once briefly during the whole day, he feels a sense of rejoicing. He also says that when he recognizes he lost it completely, he rejoices that he has the capacity to see that..."*

CATCHING VIBES

We often talk about how we catch a certain "vibe" from someone. Some people make us feel good yet others don't. This is more than a hunch or intuition, as Daniel Goleman describes in *What Makes a Leader*. He explains that the reason for this lies in the emotional center of the brain, the limbic system. The open-loop nature of this system means that how we connect with others determines our mood.

Goleman describes research where the physiology of two people in conversation is compared in a laboratory and, despite such things as heart rate and blood pressure being different at the start, within 15 minutes of conversation, the two physiological profiles become very similar. We are even affected by nonverbal expressions—the person with the strongest expression will affect the rest of the group. Goleman quotes a study by Bartel and Saavedra who found that in 70 work teams across a wide range of industries, people in meetings ended up sharing moods (both good and bad) within two hours.

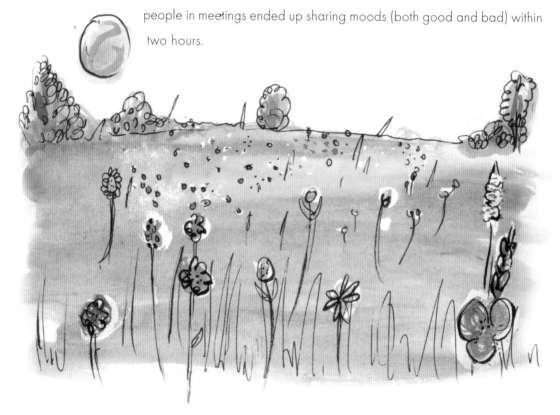

Changing Moods

When we regularly pay attention to our experience, we see how quickly moods come and go. We notice that certain moods create specific physical sensations in the body and we can tune in to our own signals and pick up early warning signs of unhelpful mood states.

Be aware that your mood is influenced by others (and vice versa). Be alert to being dragged down by the negativity of those around you. If you become used to tuning into the body through mindfulness practice, you will notice this happening and nip it in the bud through focusing on the breath, for example. What shadow does your mood cast on your colleagues? With practices such as Random Acts of Kindness (pages 98–99), we can actively create positive mood states that can be picked up by others.

THE PHYSICAL BAROMETER

Mindfulness teacher Trish Bartley developed the idea of the image of a barometer to describe the state of our moods and it is a helpful way to get a sense of perspective. This observer stance creates enough distance to prevent us from being hijacked by our emotions. Noticing that "sadness is here" or "fear is present" is not as all encompassing as saying "I am sad" or "I am afraid." We have a sense that it may be here now but it will pass, just like the weather. Regularly check in with the physical barometer of your body when you are experiencing different mood states—positive, negative, and neutral. Familiarize yourself with your own felt-sense signature of a particular mood and, by doing so, create your own early warning system.

COMMUNICATING REMOTELY

Improvements in technology have led to many of us working remotely, which presents unique challenges. When we are working and collaborating with others, we pitch our response according to the feedback we receive from them and might modify it accordingly as the conversation progresses. Due to the way our brain works, we actually begin to mirror the emotional response we see and feel in someone else.

For example, if a colleague smiles at you, your brain is activated on two levels—firstly at a motor function level that activates the neurons to make you smile back, and secondly at an emotional level that causes you to share a similar emotional response. When we are on the telephone these same mirror neurons work at an auditory level and are particularly sensitive to strong emotions (commonly negative). This mind–body social interaction is crucial. Without these types of cues we cannot connect with one another's emotional state, and it is difficult to respond appropriately when we are working together without actually being together.

The changing workplace means that we might be working from home yet communicating with colleagues and/or customers in different offices or even different parts of the world through web conferencing, conference calls, and other media. It is helpful to remember that face-to-face communication offers the most amount of information in the way of cues to each participant, as will video; audio exchanges through the telephone will offer less, and e-mail the least amount of all. Understanding this, we can modify our own behavior accordingly, for example, choosing the appropriate mode of communication according to the context. Taking the time to ease into a conference call with some social chitchat to create a more relaxed atmosphere reflects what happens in a "live" meeting and will influence what comes next.

TELEPHONE PRACTICE

The telephone ringing is a perfect cue for mindfulness practice. In the space of a ring or two there is an opportunity for you to pause, breathe, and ground yourself in the present moment. Rather than the phone call interrupting us, become available for it—and the person on the other side.

You could use a visual cue such as a colored sticker as a reminder that you intend to answer the phone in a different way.

If you sit with colleagues who expect you to answer the phone promptly or need to see that you are planning to answer the phone so they don't have to, perhaps place your hand on the phone and, if necessary, explain to them what you are doing and why.

TRY THIS

★ When the phone rings, tune into the sensations of breathing, becoming aware of the buttocks on the seat and your feet on the floor. Check in with any thoughts and emotions or physical sensations that may be present. Breathe in and breathe out.

★ Experiment—pay attention to how you feel during and after the phone call when you answer the phone in the usual way, and then do the same thing when you answer mindfully. What do you notice? Does mindfulness affect how you interact with the person on the other end?

★ Remember, too, that you can continue the practice during the conversation. Use your breath and the sensation of buttocks on the seat or feet on the floor as touchstones— pause and breathe before you speak. See Being in Conversation on page 82.

★ You can of course also do this practice before you initiate a phone call.

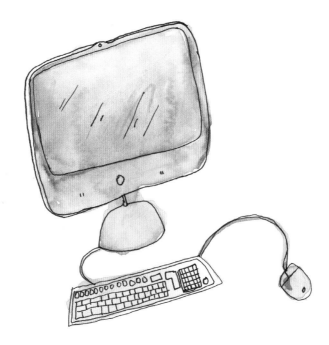

E-MAIL PRACTICE

In e-mail conversation, we are acting in isolation at each point of the exchange. An e-mail communication strips out key information that we usually receive through face-to-face or telephone exchanges. We cannot hear the tone of someone's voice or pick up on facial expressions or other body-language cues. This is further complicated by the fact that different individuals and companies follow different e-mail etiquette.

For example, if you are someone who, in e-mails, addresses colleagues by their names before stating your business, you might take offence when you receive a blunt request without any personal preamble from someone else. A request made in this way might be interpreted as a command, particularly if your mood was already low, you were feeling stressed, or had some history with the person in question.

Additional potential for misunderstanding may arise due to the global nature of today's workplace. We may be communicating with a colleague, supplier, or customer from another country whose first language differs from ours. Cultural differences influence how we communicate with others and different languages have specific conventions that can be lost in translation. A lack of awareness of this can cause offence where none was intended.

E-mails and web-conferencing are wonderful tools for connecting with others, but without awareness they also have the potential to damage relationships.

• The increase in the use of smartphones means that it has become commonplace to generate or respond to e-mails when we are on the move or our attention is elsewhere. However, multi-tasking is not always in our best interest (see page 61). When we are reading e-mails on a small screen it is harder to take in fully the content, particularly if it is complex, therefore there is a danger that we might miss something crucial.

• Tapping out an e-mail on a phone's small keyboard is not particularly easy and so we are more likely to keep exchanges short, which might be interpreted as brusque or even rude.

• The speed with which we are able to e-mail means we are more likely to react rather than respond properly, and when we communicate from a place of reaction we are not in control.

So how can we tread our way through this potential minefield without damaging professional relationships and ensure that this useful tool of global communication allows us to collaborate successfully? Practicing mindfulness can provide us with some helpful tools and there are some suggestions overleaf.

TRY THIS

⊘ Get in the habit of pausing before replying. Ask yourself: "Is now really the best time to do it?" E-mailing on the move is useful for quick replies or confirmations, but compose the more complex and sensitive e-mails when you are in a place of calm and you can give them the time and consideration that the topic and the receiver deserve. The short-term gain of a quick response may turn out to have hidden problems if the topic would have benefited from more reflection.

⊘ By regularly tuning into the body, we can pick up cues from our posture and any physical sensations we notice. These can give us important feedback about how we react to someone or certain information. Is the body tense? Where are your shoulders? What thought tone is coloring your thinking? If you are typing, how are you striking the keys—gently or with force? This body awareness is like an alarm bell warning us to wake up and be alert.

⊘ If you feel the body moving into a place of righteous indignation, irritation, or anger, wake up! If you are pounding out an e-mail response, send it to yourself or save it as a draft. When you come back and read it without the filter of emotion, you may be glad you have done so.

⊘ Think about how you are communicating with others. Put yourself in their shoes and imagine how you would feel if you received the particular e-mail you are composing. Are your words really conveying what you are trying to say or is it open to interpretation? Think about the recipient of your e-mail and, if you have an understanding of the type of e-mail they sent you, consider mirroring it—if they are chatty and asking about your weekend, respond in a similar vein.

⊘ If you are aware that you are being reactive, pause and acknowledge it. Pay attention to what you are noticing in your thoughts, emotions, and body and then take your attention to your breath or the feet on the floor. It may be helpful to remove yourself from your workstation and go for a walk to the kitchen or bathroom or have a chat with a colleague. Create some space to allow the body's natural calming response to activate. You can then respond from a different place when you are ready.

If you are taking a phone call or checking a work e-mail when you are out and about, be aware that your environment will influence your interpretation of what you are reading or hearing. If you feel that you are being interrupted, for example, you may feel annoyed or frustrated and therefore apply that emotion to the work issue where it doesn't belong. Practicing mindfulness helps us become aware of our emotions as felt sensations in the body as they arise and we become used to observing our thoughts and their particular tone (see Thought Tone, page 52). All of this adds to our awareness of the bigger picture so we are in a position to respond rather than react automatically. This awareness is generated by regularly practicing mindfulness meditation.

If we react negatively to what someone on the phone is saying, for example, we can take a moment to acknowledge how we are feeling, notice any thoughts, emotions, and physical sensations that are arising, and connect with the breath or Feet on the Floor (page 47) to activate the calming response. This pause brings us into the present moment and we have instantly moved from reaction into response mode. Our "check-in" has told us that we feel threatened and we know that when we are threatened our interpretation is more likely to be distorted. Now we can take account of that bias. We can choose how to respond appropriately (which may mean doing nothing immediately).

Remember that with auditory communication we are missing all the body language we get from face-to-face communication, and we are wired to pick up negative signals more quickly. If we can bring awareness of this to our telephone communication, we are more likely to modify what we say on the telephone to take account of this. We might deliberately engage other participants in conversation about the weekend or something light to create a particular mood before introducing a difficult topic, for example. Be alert to cues from other people in the conversation that might be interpreted in different ways, and remember that our interpretation is always influenced by our current mood.

RANDOM ACTS OF KINDNESS

Doing something kind for someone else makes us feel good and usually it makes the recipient feel good, too. We can practice random acts of kindness as a way of connecting with other people in the workplace. Moods are catching (see page 90) and so the positive vibe ripples out, touching many others, and their mood in turn influences the people they come into contact with and so it goes on.

I was reminded of this recently on a journey to work. The train driver ended his shift at a particular station and, just before the changeover, he made an announcement to wish everyone a good morning. He explained that he was going home now to his second breakfast—his first having been at 2am at the start of his shift. He told us he had enjoyed driving us and wished us well on our journey and continued talking for a minute or two. During that time the mood of the entire carriage changed. Everyone began smiling and even laughing. I could feel my own mood change from a rather dull nothing to one of lightness and connection—not just with the driver but with everyone around me.

Making Connections

Random acts of kindness can take many forms. Someone I know pays for the lunch of any member of staff who happens to be in a particular café at the same time he is. He doesn't tell them but simply settles the bill with the café owner, so when they come to pay, they are told it's already been covered. This is one way this particular manager connects with members of staff at a personal level. However, random acts of kindness need not involve money.

Kindness might take the form of a smile or wishing someone good morning, holding the door open, or helping a colleague carry some boxes. You could help explain an Excel spreadsheet to a struggling colleague, or offer someone a cup of tea or coffee. It could be doing the dishes left in the sink so the cleaner coming in at the end of the day doesn't have quite so much to do. Spending a bit of time or sharing an experience or advice costs nothing, but makes a big difference to the giver as well as the receiver.

Spread a little kindness at work today.

TRY THIS

Deliberately reach out and connect with a colleague, client, or customer. Be creative in your kindness.

- Random acts of kindness should be offered generously and without expectation of receiving something back, so let go of any element of selecting someone who "deserves it" or excluding someone who you feel doesn't.

- Random acts of kindness can be anonymous if you wish.

- Notice how it makes you feel in the moment—pay attention to the physical sensations and emotions in the body. When you reflect on your day and bring your action to mind, how do you feel now?

- Set yourself a challenge to do one random act of kindness a day.

- Notice how you feel when someone does something kind for you. Notice how it affects your mood, pay attention to any physical sensations arising and any thoughts. Notice how these feelings influence your mood and behavior, particularly with others.

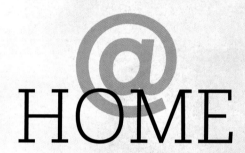

CHAPTER FOUR

HOME

We spend most of our time at work and so it is not surprising that it can begin to spill over into our own time. We can use mindfulness to stop ourselves from taking work home (physically and mentally). We can also use time and space away from work to practice more formally—learning how to sit with changing mood states, physical discomfort, and busy minds will help cultivate the skills and attitudes that we can apply to the more informal practices in the preceding chapters.

Mark's company was being bought by a much larger organization and it had been a long, drawn-out process.

"We all felt stressed and anxious about our jobs and the future. Whenever we got together that's all we could talk about—nights out became depressingly similar as the conversation always turned to work and it was always negative. I started noticing how this affected my mood —a good mood would quickly plummet after one of these events or conversations. I noticed, too, how quick I was to jump in and make my own contribution—it was as if each one of us wanted to top the other with the latest 'wrong' done to us. I realized I was contributing to my own stress and unhappiness and resolved to stop joining in. It's not easy and often I don't succeed, but it is a start and I've noticed the difference it makes to me and to my mood. When I have so little control over what is going on at work, it is good to know that my mood is one thing I can influence."

By using mindfulness, we can become aware of the role we each play in contributing to our wellbeing. Our attention is a powerful tool and through mindfulness we can learn to place it more wisely, both at work and outside working hours, allowing us to leave work where it belongs and really be at home. Our friends and family will benefit from us being with them mentally as well as physically. This time will allow our body and mind to relax—to desensitize the hair-trigger of the stress reaction—and come into a natural state of balance.

WATCHING THE BREATH

The breath is always with us and has much to tell us. When we are anxious or frightened, we usually breathe more quickly and lightly; when we are relaxed, the breath becomes longer and deeper. Regularly paying attention to the breath allows us to become familiar with our own patterns of breathing and how our state of mind affects these. Mindfulness of breathing is a core practice that can be done sitting, lying down, or standing, and even while moving. I encourage you to begin setting aside a few minutes as regularly as possible to do this practice. This will help cultivate skills that will benefit you in everyday life. Becoming familiar with the practice in the quiet of your home will make it easier when you want to draw on it in the middle of a busy day.

Although the instructions here are for a seated practice at home, watching the breath can also be done while standing in line or sitting waiting for an appointment. However, if you are doing it "out and about" there is no need to draw attention to yourself. Plant your feet on the floor, sit up tall, and begin noticing the breath (see right). You can even do it lying down in bed. You may want to read the section on how to sit comfortably on pages 42-43 for tips on how best to position yourself.

Begin by making the intention to watch your breath for just five minutes—keep it short and achievable at first, you can always continue a bit a longer if you feel like it.

TRY THIS

★ Choose an upright chair and sit with your feet firmly planted flat on the floor. Bend forward and touch your toes (as best as you can) and wriggle your buttocks to the back of the seat, then sit up. This aligns your spine so it rises naturally out of the pelvis. Place your hands in your lap or rest them on your thighs. Your eyes can be open or closed.

★ **Begin by noticing where you feel the breath most strongly at that moment.** This might be in the chest, the belly, or around the nostrils and upper lip. The actual place does not really matter, but it is helpful to make a clear intention at the start where you will be focusing your attention for the duration of your practice. Whenever your mind wanders, this is the place to come back to.

★ **Watching the breath simply means paying attention to the sensations of breathing.** Feeling the rise and fall of the chest or belly, becoming aware of that space when an in-breath turns into an out-breath and vice versa. There is no need to think about the breath or try and breathe in a particular way, although we often find that as we pay attention to our breath, it changes—and that's okay. (Sometimes watching the breath can make people more anxious—if that is the case for you, practice Feet on the Floor (see page 47) to begin with, and every so often experiment with briefly watching the breath as you may find that it gets easier after a time.)

★ In mindfulness of breathing, the breath is like an anchor—as soon as we become aware that our attention has wandered, we bring it back to the breath. When we watch our breath, we notice how active the mind is and how quickly it jumps from the breath to this, that, and something else entirely. Before we know it, in our mind, we are on vacation, somewhere warm, or perhaps we are stuck in a boardroom doing a presentation. When this occurs, the instruction is simply to notice "thinking" and, whenever the mind wanders, to bring it back. This is the practice. **The mind will wander and the practice is to bring it back, over and over again.**

Why do it?

- We can't remain stuck in rumination or thinking while paying attention to the body. Therefore, by paying attention to the breath, i.e. the body, we are naturally letting go of our thoughts (even if it is only for a few seconds). This is particularly helpful when we are caught up in some problem and can't stop thinking about it.

- We are not trying to stop our thoughts or empty our mind. Instead, **every time we become aware that we are thinking, we intentionally turn our attention toward the breath.**

- You will find that your attention is continually being pulled away by your thoughts—and that is okay. Every time you notice that you are thinking is an instance of awareness of the present moment. Every time you bring your attention back is an opportunity to strengthen those muscles of letting go.

- **Through repetition, we are strengthening the ability to disengage from our thoughts and gently bring our attention back to the present moment. By practicing regularly, we cultivate an "observer" stance that notices our experience—our thoughts, emotions, and physical sensations—as they are happening. This is helpful when something difficult arises in everyday life, as we become better able to recognize our thoughts, for example, as passing episodes rather than getting caught up in them as concrete events.**

- The more we do this in a conscious, deliberate way, the more practiced we become at turning our attention to the breath throughout the day.

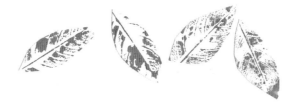

• Through constant practice, the breath becomes an anchor—turning our attention to it in moments of crisis, we instantly draw on our practice.

• When we watch the breath, we notice how our experience is always changing. Our attention is constantly pulled away by thoughts or the itch at the end of the nose. We become more at ease with perpetual change and recognize that it is part and parcel of experience, rather than something to be feared. We learn to let go of trying to control our experience and, instead, allow it take us in unexpected and unlooked-for directions.

TIPS

★ Do this as regularly as you can—it is better to do a shorter practice more often than a longer practice only every once in a while.

★ Choose a specific time, for example when you get up, come in from work, or before you go to bed and stick to it. If you can make it part of your daily routine, you are more likely to keep it up.

★ It can be helpful to repeat silently to yourself "in—out" on each in- and out-breath.

★ Be patient and gentle with yourself. Everyone's mind wanders (and will always do so). When I first started practicing, I would close my eyes and two minutes later open them again, sure that at least 30 minutes had passed! You will find that it becomes easier, so gradually extend the time period if you like.

★ If you are worried about time, set an alarm (perhaps muffle it under a cushion so as not to startle yourself). There are also numerous free meditation timers for phones and computers available on the Internet.

WATCHING THE BREATH
AND THE BODY

As you become familiar with watching the breath, you can extend the practice to include awareness of the body. Turning our attention to physical sensations arising in the body is a way of tuning in and acknowledging what we are feeling. We may notice subtle physical sensations, such as a sense of pressure or cloth against skin; maybe a sense of temperature. Or perhaps we experience a sense of lightness, tightness, or agitation in a particular part of the body, and become aware of how these relate to particular thoughts and emotions.

Why do it?

- We practice staying with minor discomforts, as they are a safe way to practice staying with sensations that we don't like. Then, if and when we experience emotional or physical pain or discomfort, we will have already developed skills to be with these to some degree.

- Staying with uncomfortable sensations (however briefly) may feel counter-intuitive, but it is different from the usual ignoring, distracting, or numbing out, which we do too often with alcohol, drugs (prescription or otherwise), or other unhealthy activities such as overwork. Learning to act differently is an important step in accepting our experience, even if we wish it were different.

- Keeping unwanted emotions at bay creates tension and tightness in the body —and we literally stiffen up. Not only is this exhausting in the moment of resistance, but the tension can create health issues.

- Acceptance allows us to be with our difficulties. Just as you exercise to tone the body's muscles to develop physical strength, developing these skills when we are well means that we can draw on them in times of trouble. The body will give us invaluable feedback if we are able to be aware of it.

TRY THIS

- Begin with Feet on the Floor (see page 47), followed by a short period of Watching the Breath (see page 102).

- When you feel ready, expand your awareness to include the whole body. The breath is still there but it is no longer taking center stage; instead, it is just part of the background, like a radio playing in a nearby room.

- Become aware of any physical sensations arising. Notice whether there is a sense of resistance towards them or maybe a feeling of "ahh, that's nice." We are not looking for any particular experience but simply noticing whatever is there (and there may well be nothing).

- Even if no internal sensations arise, we can often become aware of how our body feels in contact with the floor or chair—a sense of connection and touch. In your mind's eye, scan around the body and notice any instances of this. What does that place feel like? What do you notice?

- Remember that the breath is part of the body, so at any time there is the option of becoming aware of the sensations of breathing.

- If a particular sensation, such as an itch, is clamoring for your attention, you have choices about what to do next. First notice where it is. You can focus your attention on the breath, noticing the in- and the out-breath, while maintaining awareness of the itch. Alternatively, you can direct the breath into the itch (or whatever the discomfort may be) and imagine the breath entering and leaving the body through that point. Finally, if it feels okay, you can be curious about the itch—exploring it with a sense of interest rather than analysis. Is it constant or changing? Moving around or static? Remember that we are not trying to get rid of—or change—the sensation, but rather, we are practicing being with it in a different way. If there are strong feelings of discomfort, it is always okay to move. **You should never sit through pain or discomfort with gritted teeth. Instead, make a deliberate decision to move and then adjust your position with mindful awareness.**

- Finish by narrowing your attention back onto the breath for a few minutes.

BEING WITH THOUGHTS

One of the commonest misconceptions about meditation is that we are trying to empty our mind and stop thinking. Another is that "my mind is too busy to meditate." Both of these spotlight the issue that many of us have with our thoughts—the constant nattering in the background, sometimes badgering, occasionally hectoring, quite often mean and judgmental—our thoughts are like a hydrant left spewing water from a never-ending source.

We will never be able to stop our thoughts, so we might as well give up trying to avoid them. Try it now – stop thinking! What do you notice? It takes a huge amount of effort and we are immediately measuring how we are doing, and of course that is thinking too, so we try and stop that and are quickly caught up in a pretzel of contradictions. So the suggestion is to relax—let go of trying to stop your thoughts and, in fact, invite them in. This is harder than it sounds, so it is worth practicing this during a sitting practice from time to time.

When we pay attention to our thoughts we don't want to get caught up in them or start to analyze them, but it can be helpful to notice the content. This is feedback about where your attention currently is, as well as feedback on your mood and general wellbeing. Noticing our thoughts tells us what is preying on our mind. Being able to be aware of our thoughts simply as feedback rather than fact gives us an opportunity to pick up warning signs that might be skewing our judgment or affecting our performance. When we are aware of our experience we have the opportunity to take wise action.

TRY THIS

Take the time to set yourself up in sitting practice as described in Breath and Body (see page 106). After settling your attention on the breath and body, invite your thoughts to take center stage. This is often when we notice our thoughts get stage fright and disappear into the wings, although inevitably, after a while, they begin to creep back. You can try any of the following, although I would recommend choosing just one to focus on during each session.

★ In this practice we are seeing our thoughts simply as thoughts—like clouds in the sky. Some are dark and heavy, others wispy, some move really fast but others hang around and are hard to shift. Noticing the quality of the thought can be helpful.

★ Name that tune! If it's one of your top 10 tunes (see page 75), identify it.

★ Some thoughts are stickier than others. When this happens, acknowledge it and take your attention to the breath, breathe in and out while holding that sticky thought in awareness. By giving your attention another job to do, we can move it from the thought and yet not suppress the thought. We are simply using the breath to *be* with the thought.

★ If you find visualizations helpful, you can imagine yourself by a stream or river and picture yourself placing an individual thought on a leaf and pushing it off into the current. Sometimes the thought leaf might spin around a bit or get caught up in other leaves, but eventually the current will pick it up and take it away.

★ You can try counting your thoughts. When you lose count, go back to one.

★ Labeling your thoughts as thinking or planning or rumination can be helpful (see pages 72–73).

★ Remember that we are not interested in the content of thoughts. They are simply passing objects that momentarily catch our attention. Our thoughts are influenced by the mood we are in, so they cannot be relied upon as facts. Reminding ourselves that thoughts are not facts can be really helpful.

MAKING FRIENDS WITH OURSELVES AND OTHERS

There is a traditional practice called Loving Kindness, which is done to cultivate and draw out feelings of kindness, connection, empathy, and kinship, which are very different from romantic or sentimental love. When we practice Loving Kindness, the area of the brain that involves motivation becomes active. Motivation drives our intentions and intention drives our behavior, so Loving Kindness practices can be very powerful at transforming our behavior. This is commonly done as a sitting practice, so it is one to do at home.

We do this practice without any expectation of feeling a particular emotion. We are not looking for a warm fuzzy feeling. In fact, this practice is one where we may experience a certain amount of resistance. **This practice is not about changing other people or expecting anything in return from others.** The practice is about cultivating and drawing out qualities that are present in every one of us but it can take time to notice a difference.

Research in a randomized-control trial showed that practicing Loving Kindness once a week produced increases in daily expressions of positive emotions that in turn fueled a wide range of personal resources, such as increased mindfulness, a greater sense of purpose in life, and social support, among others. These, in turn, increased a person's overall sense of life satisfaction as well as positive emotions, particularly when interacting with others.

When you try Loving Kindness practice, avoid judging it or expecting particular things from it. Just do it and see what happens. This is a good practice for all of us to do as many of us treat ourselves too harshly. It is advisable to begin offering loving kindness to someone you care, about before introducing yourself "through the back door."

MAKING FRIENDS WITH YOURSELF

Begin by taking the time to settle yourself by spending a period of time doing Breath and Body (see page 106). It is really important never to leave this stage out as it grounds us in the present moment—creating an inner stability that is useful in the later stages. Remember that you can return to the anchor of the breath if things feel difficult at any time.

- Bring to mind someone you care about—it might be a teacher, mentor, friend, a family member, or even a much-loved pet. Someone who, when you think of them, gives you a sense of an internal smile or opening towards them.

- Bring your chosen person to mind and then repeat silently to yourself the following phrases May you be healthy. May you be happy. May you be free from suffering (see page 113).

- The phrases are simply conduits of attention, so feel free to adapt them to whatever resonates with you, although short and simple is easiest. Allow each phrase some space and then hear it resonate in the mind and body. We are not expecting to feel anything at all. Repeat these phrases perhaps two or three times.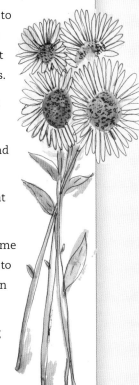

- Then, bring yourself to mind alongside this person you care about and repeat the phrases but using "may we…".

- Once again pay attention to those moments when you notice a resistance and those moments you lean into and want more of.

- Then, letting go of the person you care about (for now), picture yourself and repeat the phrases but using "may I…".

- Pay attention to what resonates within you. It is quite common to notice some resistance. We might feel unworthy or perhaps it feels selfish to direct attention to ourselves. However, it is worth remembering that if we look after our own wellbeing, we will be in a better position to look after those we care about.

- If these phrases do feel difficult, simply go back to the previous stage, picturing yourself alongside the person you care about and using "we."

- End by expanding the circle to include the person we care about, ourselves, and any other close family or friends.

Making Friends with Others

There are often people at work whom we find difficult. This might be because of a particular history we might have with them, but sometimes we just don't warm to them. We can do Loving Kindness practice for a person like this and we do it to transform *our* attitude to them. We are reminding ourselves that this person is a human being like us—someone's son or daughter, perhaps a mother or father, brother or sister, someone who wants to be happy just like we do, someone who wants to be free from pain and suffering.

Notice what you have in common (even at its simplest—the fact that you work together or the color of your hair or eyes), as well as anything positive about them or good they have done for you or others. It is important to remember that we are not trying to change them in any way, but rather create a shift in our attitude towards them. We are not condoning anything they might have done either.

When you are trying practices like this, begin with someone who is perhaps a bit annoying, but if, at any time, it feels too much, return to Making Friends with Yourself on the previous page. It is important not to try this with anyone who has done you a great hurt in any way.

Follow the instructions on page 111 and, after you have taken the time to be with the breath and body, move into doing Loving Kindness for someone you care about, and then for yourself *before* bringing to mind the person who is causing you difficulties at work. Remember to use the breath as an anchor at any time if you need to. Picture this person and then repeat the following phrases or your own variations:

May you be healthy. May you be happy. May you be free from suffering.

Notice how the words resonate with you. If you do feel a resistance to any particular words, play around with them—sometimes changing the words can make a difference. For example, if wishing someone to be happy feels too difficult, perhaps you could wish that they "be free from anger." Experiment and test words and notice how your body responds by being aware of physical sensations. When you find some words or phrases that feel right for you, repeat them silently in the same way as before.

End the practice in the same way as on page 111 (repeating the phrases for a round or two). End with a few minutes focusing solely on the breath.

SOME POSSIBLE PHRASES

May I / We / You be...

PEACEFUL   CALM   HAPPY   HEALTHY   SAFE   WELL

PROTECTED FROM HARM   AT EASE WITH MY LIFE   HAVE PEACE OF MIND

May I / We / You be free from...

JEALOUSY   ANGER   PAIN   WORRY   SUFFERING

MINDFUL BREAKFAST

Every morning, I prepare a fruit and vegetable juice for breakfast. People often ask me how I find the time, but juicing has become a mini mindfulness practice for me and is simply part of my morning routine. As I wash the earth off the produce, there is a sense of where it came from—the rain, sun, and cold helping it to grow, the people who picked it and sent it to the city. I chop the vegetables knowing that I'm chopping the vegetables—I focus on the task at hand, rather than thinking about the day to come. A friend who juices, too, often comes to mind, and there is a momentary connection, like an internal smile, as the activity joins us together. When the juice is made, I set it aside and clean everything before drinking it—the whole process takes about ten minutes. I rarely feel rushed, even if I'm running late, as I allow myself simply to be where I am.

What is your breakfast routine? Do you stop long enough to nourish yourself? If you do eat breakfast, how do you eat it? Are you reading the newspaper, checking your work e-mails, or making sure the children have everything they need for school? We all lead busy lives and, if children are involved, breakfast can often feel like a battleground, but if that is the case, how does that make you feel?

Experiment and observe the differences between your normal routine and a breakfast routine that incorporates mindfulness. Make a decision which you prefer. Even if it is not possible to do this every day, perhaps it is possible to do it once a week or at the weekend?

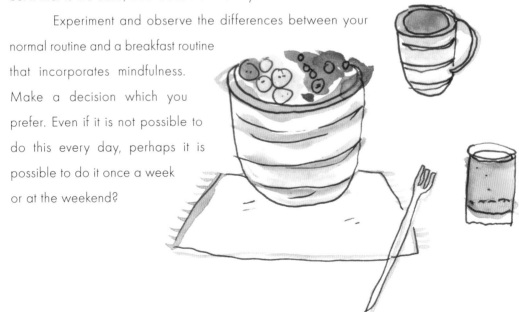

TRY THIS

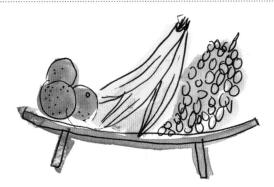

★ For a few days, pay attention to your breakfast routine. Notice what you do and how you do it. Notice how you feel immediately afterwards. If you haven't eaten breakfast at home, do you pick something up on the way to work and, if so, what is it? Perhaps you eat breakfast at work, how does that feel?

★ Now make an intention to eat your breakfast mindfully. Remember that any activity can be done mindfully by intentionally paying attention to what you are doing without judging it. When you notice thoughts intruding, simply bring your attention back to preparing or eating your food. Food is more than just taste—explore what you are doing with all your senses—the colors and textures, as well as the smell. Savor them.

★ If you are eating breakfast at work, you can still eat it mindfully. It might not be ideal but if that's all that is possible for you to do at this point, then that is good enough. Start where you are.

★ It is a misconception that we need more time to do an activity mindfully. What can happen though is that when we become interested in the activity, we slow down and linger over it longer than we normally would. So perhaps allow yourself the luxury of a bit of extra time to do this, if possible.

★ As before, notice how you feel during the activity and immediately afterwards.

★ Compare the two ways of eating breakfast, and, if you have found it helpful, explore how you can introduce mindfulness into your everyday breakfast routine.

THE JOURNEY

They say that it's the journey, not the destination, that is important. Every day we travel to work —on foot, in cars, by train, ferry or bus—and often that journey is something we endure. Notice your regular journey—pay attention to it and become aware of any thoughts and emotions arising and how the body responds to these. How do you feel when you arrive at work—calm and relaxed or stressed and anxious? People often say to me that they don't want to pay attention as their journeys are awful, so why bother? However, shutting down your experience comes at a price. It can become a habitual response to situations that we find unpleasant— and unfortunately also to the pleasant encounters—as opening ourselves up to these experience is an all-or-nothing attitude. By repeatedly shutting down, you are closing yourself off from life. How can we do things differently?

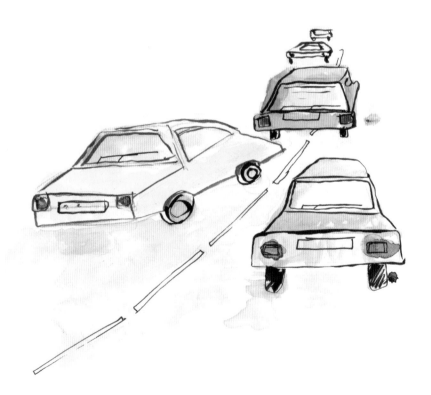

Your Time in the Car, Bus, or Train

Be creative about how you can bring mindfulness into your journey—remember that all you have to do is deliberately pay attention to your experience without judging it and without wanting any particular outcome. Experiment and notice how you feel during your journey and how it affects you for the rest of the day.

Commuting by train or bus can result in being crammed up against other bodies to a degree that is far too close for comfort. It is not pleasant, so acknowledge what you are feeling. Notice whether you are holding your breath—relax and let go. Notice whether the body is tensed as you maintain your "space" against possible intruders—let go. Become aware of the feet on the floor, the buttocks on the seat (if you are lucky enough to be sitting). Breathe in your discomfort while staying grounded and strong. It is important to recognize that **we are not trying to make our experience pleasant or better, we are simply being with it as it is**. Try it and see what happens.

Traveling by car gives us our own space, but our journey can still be interrupted by other drivers, cutting us off or clogging up the roads and causing jams. Make the intention that your car journey will be your practice. Turn off the radio or music and allow yourself to be with the sounds around you. Open the window to smell the air, be it pleasant or not. Feel the steering wheel beneath your hands and, when the lights change to red, brake and breathe. Follow the breath until they change to green. Do the same at the next traffic light. How do you feel when you arrive?

Arriving when You Arrive

Commuters are often at the mercy of cancelled or delayed trains or buses or traffic jams. We know we are supposed to be somewhere else, so the news that we are going to be late or miss our appointment can cause anger and frustration that we then carry with us for the rest of the journey, and often well into our day. Instead, **notice the emotions as they arise**-pay attention to where you feel them in the body. There may be a sense of tension or stiffness in the neck or shoulders, perhaps a rolling sensation in the belly. **Turn your attention to the body with a spirit of curiosity to see what's there.** You may not feel any sensations at all but it is the act of tuning in that is important.

Notice any stories that are arising around being late-blame, judgment, worry, anxiety. Are you taking that anger and frustration out on those around you-the ticket collector, the fellow passenger pushing in front of you? **Name any emotions that you are aware of and then, holding on to these emotions and sensations, focus on the breath:** breathing in and breathing out. Remind yourself that there is nothing you can do. You will arrive when you arrive. Let go of any negative stories as they are simply fuelling the fire of frustration.

Turn off Autopilot

When we perform the same action repeatedly, we begin to operate on automatic pilot. We get from A to B but without any real awareness of what our experience actually was. We can wake ourselves by doing something different. Can you vary your journey from time to time? Perhaps walk all or part the way, take a different route, travel by train instead of car or vice versa. When we do something different, the body wakes up, the senses become alert, and we notice so much more. We arrive at our destination feeling alert. You may not be able to do this all the time, but do it when you can.

Connecting with Others

Many faceless people help us on our daily journey. Some we may see regularly, such as the ticket collector, the toll-booth operator—familiar faces without a name—but others work behind the scenes and often through the night to make sure we get to where we need to be on time. As you travel, make a deliberate intention to notice these people. Make eye contact, say thank you or good morning. **Connect with your fellow travelers**. You don't have to strike up a conversation, but be aware of all the other people going about their day—like you, each one of them just wants to be happy, but there may be all kinds of difficulties going on in their lives. Silently wish them well on your journey.

Traveling on Foot

Walking is a great activity to do if your mind is busy and being outside connects us with the natural world. To walk mindfully, walk knowing that you are walking (take out your earphones). There is no need to walk slowly, simply pay attention to your body—the air on your face, the sensations of your feet touching the ground, the breath entering and leaving the body. Widen your attention out to include the environment, and then bring it back to focus just on the feet and the body.

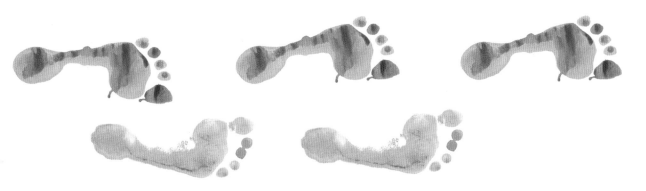

TECHNOLOGY DETOX

Staying connected with the workplace when we are out and about can be helpful. However, we can become a slave to our BlackBerry or smartphone too easily. This is particularly true during out-of-office hours or while on vacation. We may think that just "checking in" has little impact, but every time we do so we are turning our attention towards work. When we are mentally "at work" we are not present, wherever that might be. This impacts negatively on whoever we are with as well as on ourselves.

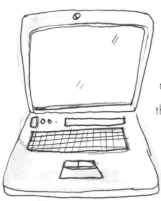

I have noticed that when I am feeling stressed or anxious, I repeatedly check in with work. I became aware of a driven quality to this action. Then I noticed what happened next. If there was nothing new, a story might arise about why not; or there may be a message that required action that I might or might not be able to take. This had an immediate effect on me physically and emotionally and could then easily affect my mood for the rest of the day.

Switching Off

Noticing the negative impact, I decided to try an experiment. First, I tried telling myself not to look at work e-mails outside of work, but unfortunately lack of self-control meant that was unsuccessful. Next, I changed the settings so I could temporarily remove my work e-mail from my phone. Now, if I wanted to check e-mails, it had to be a deliberate choice rather than an unconscious action. The first few times I felt a frisson of anxiety, but these moments gradually grew further and further apart and I noticed that when I did go back to work, I felt as if I'd really been away. Now I turn off my work e-mail at the end of the working day as a matter of course and perform better on my return as a result of it.

Often our behavior has become so habitual that our experience seems normal. We can't remember when it might have been different. If this is the case for you try the following experiment.

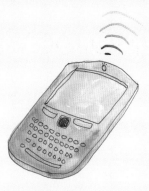

- Decide when you can legitimately and reasonably expect to be "off duty" and make an intention to reclaim this time for yourself.

- Change the settings on your phone to turn off or remove a particular e-mail account. Some phones can be set up to do this automatically at a set time each day.

- Let colleagues know that when you are on holiday or out of the office, you won't be checking e-mails or available for phone calls. If there is resistance to this, negotiate a time-limited period during which you will check in.

- Pay attention to your experience—notice any sensations of "wanting" or "resistance." Notice how your mood is affected as well as any effects on those around you.

- Be prepared to experience some resistance from yourself (as well as others) to this, but be persistent and stick it out. If you are struggling, begin with shorter periods, such as evenings and weekends.

- Notice how you feel when you return to the office after giving yourself a technology detox.

BACK-TO-WORK BLUES

Even just thinking about going back to work after a weekend or a vacation can bring down our mood and we often find ourselves projecting forward to the workdays ahead while we are still on our own time. This "future thinking" is unhelpful as it is pulling us away from being in the present moment. Although we may physically be with our children in the park, out with friends, or cuddling up to a loved one on the sofa, we are not present mentally. This stops us enjoying these precious moments. It is also detrimental to our relationships as people feel unloved or undervalued and relegated to below the workplace. We know when the person we are with is distracted and not paying attention to us, and if this is your default behavior at home the consequences can be devastating.

People sometimes tell me that they check their work e-mails on Sunday night so that "there are no surprises on Monday morning." However, as soon as you log on and turn your attention to work, your mind will become engaged in whatever is going on

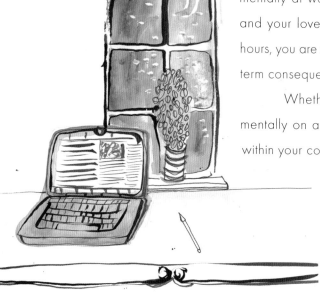

there. Time off is meant to be time away from the pressures and demands of work, so if you are mentally at work, you are short-changing yourself and your loved ones. By extending your working hours, you are more vulnerable to stress and its long-term consequences (see page 28).

Whether you choose to go to work mentally on a Sunday night is up to you, but it is within your control to do something different.

TRY THIS

★ When you are on vacation or it's the weekend—really be off work. Give yourself the gift of temporarily setting to one side the weight of work. When you find your mind wandering to work issues, gently bring it back to whatever you are doing and know what you are doing while you are doing it, whether that is reading a story to your children, visiting an elderly parent, choosing the veg for the Sunday dinner, going for a walk, or spending time with friends.

★ If you have gotten into the habit of checking e-mails on a Sunday night, pay attention to how this activity affects you in terms of your thinking, your emotions, and what you feel physically in the body. Acknowledge how it makes you feel emotionally. It is only until you bring something into awareness that you can do it differently. Make a clear intention to break the habit (and be gentle with yourself when you forget). It can be helpful to engage family members in reminding you of your intention when you are tempted to log on. Notice what drives you—that automatic moment when you find yourself steering towards your computer, what do you notice if you pay attention to your experience? What do you notice afterwards—where are your thoughts going?

★ If you find your mind becoming busy and your mood lowering at the prospect of work the next day, practice mindfulness. Try a Mindful Minute (see page 54) if you are in the middle of something, or Feet on the Floor (see page 47), or a Breathing space (see page 78). If you have time, do one of the longer practices such as Watching the Breath on page 102.

DARING TO BE A BEGINNER

When we are children, we learn new things all the time. Every new experience and skill stretches us, gives us confidence, and widens our world. However, as adults our learning often slows right down or even grinds to a halt.

As we become good at particular skills we may specialize and even become an expert. As an expert we may feel we have a certain position to uphold and so we may be reluctant to jeopardize our status. Whether we are an expert or not, as adults we are often self-conscious and worried about making a fool of ourselves, therefore our default is not to do anything that is outside of our comfort zone.

Research has shown that the brain is much more plastic than previously thought and the potential for learning new things is always there, "use it or lose it" is just as applicable to the brain as to the physical body. So there is a physiological rationale for learning new skills, as well as a psychological one. If our life revolves entirely around work and our identity is defined by what we do, we become more vulnerable when things go wrong at work. Our very being is shaken.

However, if we can expand our interests and include non-work-related activities, we are building our confidence. It might seem scary and we may be anxious and nervous, but it is only when we move out of our comfort zone that we are going to grow. When we realize that we can do something even when we feel apprehensive at first, we realize that perhaps we can do other things, too. Learning new skills through different activities often brings us into contact with a different circle of people. This brings with it an opportunity to talk about non-work-related things and so *really* give ourselves a break.

- Learning something as an adult is a totally different experience from learning at school—you can study purely out of interest without an agenda. You could learn DIY or plumbing, sewing or cooking, a foreign language or art appreciation. You could learn fencing, squash, or swimming, woodcarving or how to play the harmonica—the possibilities are endless.

- Having a regular class gives you a reason to leave work on time. Regularly working overtime is not good for your health. You may be tired, but using your mind or body differently is relaxing in its own way.

- Participating in certain activities, such as singing in a choie, actually reduces stress as we do them.

- Physical activities are often stress busters. Kickboxing will give a healthy release to any stress hormones built up during the day. Qigong, tai chi, or yoga are also activities that focus on the body—and remember that when we focus on the body we get out of the head. However, any physical activity can be done mindfully—simply pay attention to your experience as it unfolds without judging it.

- If the weather permits, spend time outside as being outdoors (even in the city) connects you to the passing seasons and natural world that gives us a wider perspective.

- Learning a new skill requires paying attention and focus so this is a great way to switch off the work-mind.

- Give yourself permission to be a beginner—letting go of any expectations or agenda. Is there something you've always yearned to do? What would you like to try and learn?

SOUND VERSUS NOISE

We perform best when we are focused, and yet we have many distractions to contend with at work. One of the most difficult can be working within a noisy environment, particularly if your office is open plan, therefore it can be helpful to practice allowing a distraction such as a noise, judged as unpleasant, simply to be a sound.

According to The Oxford Dictionary, noise is "a sound, especially one that is loud or unpleasant or that causes disturbance," whereas sound is "vibrations that travel through the air or another medium and can be heard when they reach a person's or animal's ear." Which one sounds more unpleasant and something that you would avoid?

We talk about the sound of birdsong but the noise of drilling—the descriptive words we choose contain an element of judgment. When we judge something as unpleasant, we mentally move away from it, our body tenses up against it, and all our defenses go up. This takes up a lot of energy and creates tension in the body that can quickly become habitual, causing long-term health problems.

If we can practice being with noise as sound, we can transfer those skills to everyday situations at work where the environment may challenge our attention and stir up emotions, such as irritation and frustration. These can then ripple out and affect others, our performance, as well as our overall sense of well-being. Instead, the constant ringing of telephones or the drilling going on outside simply becomes a combination of pitch, tone, and timbre. We can allow it to rise and pass by without getting hooked into it. We can use the breath to anchor ourselves if we feel strong emotions arising.

TRY THIS

· Find a time and a place where you can sit for a short period of time. The length of time is your choice.

· Take the time to find a comfortable posture (see page 42) and spend a few minutes settling your attention on the breath in the place where you can feel it most strongly (see page 102).

· When you feel ready, widen your awareness from the breath to include sounds. These might be sounds near or far away.

· Notice when you judge a sound as pleasant or unpleasant—what sensations do you notice in the body when you judge a sound as "noise?"

· Become aware of any story or label you attach to a sound. When you become aware of it, simply let it go as a thought and bring your attention back to the breath before widening out once again.

· We are receiving sound—it passes through the air, reaches us, and then continues on its way. It is not personal. There is no need to create a story around it. Sounds are simply vibrations within the air we breathe.

· Allow your whole body to act as a radar, receiving any sound that comes your way. There's no need to hunt for sound—noticing the sound of silence in the periods when it arises. What is the sound of silence? How silent is the absence of sound?

· Sounds are like our thoughts. They appear whether we want them to or not and we have no control over them. We can choose, however, how we respond to them. We don't need to become attached to them or construct a convoluted story around them. We will do both of these things, but when we realize we are doing so, we can let go.

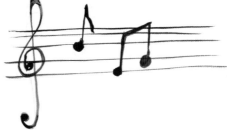

SITTING WITH UPSET

Emotional upset is the most powerful distraction to attention. How we feel is important to us so the brain will always make any unhappiness a high priority. Consequently, if we are upset, we will find it difficult to concentrate as our attention is hijacked by our thoughts, which can very quickly spiral into rumination as we try to solve our emotional "problem."

The more we strengthen our ability to let go, i.e. by constantly returning to a point of focus when we get distracted, the easier we will find it to let go when we are upset. Therefore, any practice that helps us improve letting go and keeps us from coming back over and over again is going to benefit us. However, there will also be occasions when we are caught up in emotions and we want to do something positive about it but don't know what or how.

Before you try this, it is important to have some experience of sitting and watching the breath and body (see pages 102-107). We need to have honed the skill of using the breath as an anchor and practiced unhooking our attention from our thoughts. It is important to have gotten used to tuning into the body and paying attention to physical sensations as they arise. We want to have practiced using our attention like a flashlight—sometimes keeping it focused and other times widening it out to shine a light on our experience and beyond. Develop these skills before trying this practice.

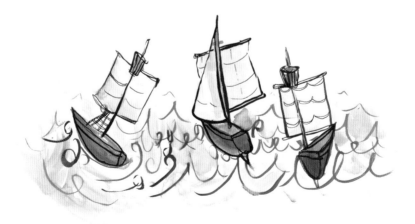

TRY THIS

★ Settle yourself into your seat (see page 102) and spend as much time as you need resting the attention on the breath. Feel the sensations of breath and body and use them as an anchor—this is how we prevent ourselves from being swept away by strong emotions.

★ When you feel ready, allow your attention to expand to include whatever is going on for you, while at the same time maintaining your attention on the body. Notice how what you are feeling emotionally is playing out in terms of physical sensations in the body. Name any emotions that you become aware of and explore where you are feeling them in the body. Direct the breath into that part of the body if it feels helpful.

★ Become aware of your thoughts—what stories are playing out in your head? Remind yourself that our thoughts are not facts but simply passing states of mind, like the weather.

★ If it is helpful, you can visualize yourself at the top of the waterfall—standing or sitting close to the edge, but in a place of safety. Allow yourself to feel a sense of connection with the ground. Your thoughts are like the water rushing by—some of them are so strong that you get "soaked" by them, some of them get stuck in little eddies around the rocks and hang around for a while, but all of them eventually tumble out of your field of vision. You remain safe at the top—watching them go but not getting swept away by them.

★ Regularly bring your attention back to the breath and the body. To prevent you getting hijacked by your thoughts and emotions, we may focus mostly on the breath and body and only spend a second or two turning toward the difficult emotions. This dance between the two is a safe way to allow ourselves to be with a strong emotion.

★ Finish by focusing solely on the breath.

When you do this practice, remember that we are not trying to make the difficult feelings go away. If you experience strong feelings while at work, acknowledge how you are feeling and ground yourself with Feet on the Floor (see page 47).

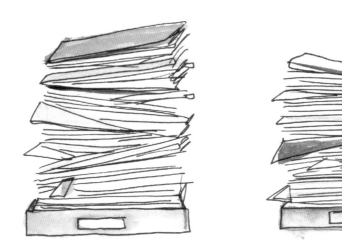

BRINGING YOUR WORK HOME

Taking work home doesn't always just mean physical work. How often do you find yourself going over and over something that has happened at work? What work are you bringing home in your head? Perhaps it is an argument you had with a colleague or your boss, maybe you made a mistake, or perhaps it's about a piece of work you have been laboring over to get "just right." It is more than likely to be something that has upset you, and it becomes difficult to let it go. You might find yourself replaying the scenario over and over, analyzing it from different angles, trying to second-guess what others were thinking or possible consequences. These are the thoughts that often keep us awake at night or make us feel stressed, anxious, and irritable.

The mind/body connection is so strong that every time we bring an upsetting scenario to mind, it as if we are experiencing it again. The thoughts are perceived as a threat and the fight or flight response is activated and maintained by our thinking (see page 22). We may find our body has a strong physical reaction to this mental "perceived threat"—faster breathing, nausea, sweaty palms, an urge to empty the bowels. These sensations are unpleasant and so thoughts arise around them—why do I feel like this? I shouldn't feel like this These sort of thoughts act as a feedback loop, keeping the stress response activated. How should we handle this?

The priority is to turn our attention to the body—to the physical sensations of our experience. It is simplest to focus on a strong sensation initially, this may be something like the weight of your buttocks on the chair if you are seated, or the sensations of your feet on the floor. Explore the point of contact, becoming aware of any sensations of temperature, texture, or weight.

Expand your attention gradually, including the whole body. Become aware of the breath, any internal sensations arising, the impact of the external environment—a breeze on the cheek, a smell. Be curious about your experience without any agenda.

The more we practice mindfulness through sitting meditation (see pages 102–107), the more practiced we become at picking up the early signs that we are falling into a pattern of unhelpful thinking. At the first sign of this, particularly if it is a habitual thought, **turn your attention to the body to nip it in the bud**. It is a discipline that will break the cycle and help desensitize the stress response. The more you allow yourself to get caught up in unhelpful thinking, the more you reinforce it. It is within your power to shift your attention away, but it is hard, so be patient and just keep doing it at every opportunity.

It is important to let go of any expectation that mindfulness will make the unpleasantness disappear. As soon as this agenda creeps in, it sabotages the practice. **We practice mindfulness without expectations of achieving a particular outcome.** We are simply being with our experience (even if we don't like it), and paradoxically, this acceptance becomes transformative so while the unpleasantness does not necessarily go away because we are not reacting to it, it feels a lot less difficult.

Be curious about your experience without any agenda

TIRED LEGS OR ANXIOUS MIND?

Gravity is a stressor and so it's no wonder that often our legs are tired at the end of the day, particularly if we have been on our feet for many hours. This traditional yoga pose is a great restorative and you can do it for as little as five minutes to feel the benefit. As well as rejuvenating tired legs, Legs-Up-the-Wall can calm the anxious mind, help with insomnia, and gently stretch out the back of the legs, front torso, and the back of the neck. It is a helpful pose to do at the end of the day.

You will need a clear wall space to rest your legs against, a mat or blanket if the floor is uncarpeted, and one or two thick folded blankets or a firm bolster. A weighted eye bag placed over the eyes once you are in the pose may be appreciated. Notice whether there is a sense of "I should be able to..." popping into the mind and remind yourself that we always start from where we are at. There is absolutely no expectation of our legs having to be perfectly flat against the wall.

The traditional yoga pose, Viparita Karani, is a great restorative.

Caution Some teachers advise that women avoid even gentle inverted poses during menstruation. You should definitely avoid this if you have any serious eye problems, such as glaucoma. If you have any neck or back problems, only do this under supervision of an experienced teacher.

LEGS-UP-THE-WALL

1 To begin, take off your shoes. Your height and flexibility will determine where you position your folded blankets or bolster. If you are less flexible, place your support further away from the wall and keep it lower. If you are more flexible, use a higher support closer to the wall. If you are shorter, move closer. However, as always, experiment and discover what works best for you.

2 Position your support about a hand's width from the wall, then, sitting sideways, on an out-breath, gently swing your legs up against the wall and lower your back, shoulders, and head to the floor. It may take a few attempts and you might need to move the support around until you feel comfortable.

3 You want your chin to be lower than your forehead, so rest your head on a cushion if necessary. We are looking for a gentle arch of the torso over your support. Keep your legs relaxed but firm.

4 Your arms can be at your sides with your palms upwards or, if your mind is very busy, rest your palms on the belly.

5 Place an eye bag over your eyes if you like. Take a few moments to soften into the floor and allow yourself to be supported by the floor. Rest your attention on the breath, feeling the sensations of breathing, the belly rising and falling. Every out–breath becomes a release, a softening, a letting go of thoughts, tension, and fatigue as you rest in the present moment.

6 When you are ready to come down (after 5–15 minutes), gently slide off the support before lowering your legs and resting on your side for a few breaths. Then come into sitting. Feel free to end this pose early, particularly if it is uncomfortable.

WAKEFUL NIGHTS

Lying awake at night can be stressful. We might wake up thinking about work and then thoughts about being awake intrude and start a spiral of anxiety. The easiest way to disengage the thinking mind is to turn our attention to the body. It is important to let go of wishing for a particular outcome. Remind yourself that by doing any of the three practices here you are resting the mind, and if the mind rests, the body rests.

PRACTICE ONE

★ Lie on your back with your feet falling apart and become aware of the body in contact with the bed. Perhaps begin by scanning the body from the heels all the way up along the legs, buttocks, the back, neck, and head. Just notice how the body is held and supported by the bed. Allow yourself to be supported. Let go of any sense of "holding on." Take a deep breath in and let it out.

★ Place one or both hands on your belly and drop your attention to the palms of the hand. Become aware of the contact of the hand with the belly and begin to become aware of the breath, and in particular the out-breath. You may find it helpful to say "out-breath" silently to yourself each time you become aware of it, the hand gently falling as the belly contracts and the breath leaves the body. Notice how the body responds to each out-breath. Allow the body to let go of the out-breath completely.

★ Just continue watching the breath in this way. After a while, you may find yourself watching both the in- and the out-breath equally and that's fine.

★ If, at any time, thoughts intrude about "not falling asleep" or work-related issues, just label them as thinking, gently remind yourself that you are simply breathing without any expectation of falling asleep, and escort your attention back to the out-breath (we can do this over and over again). Regardless of whether you do fall asleep or not, being with the breath in this way will settle the mind and you will feel more rested.

Tips

There are some practical things you can try to help aid sleep. As with all these practices, experiment and discover what you notice when you try different things.

- Avoid bringing your work phone into the bedroom. That winking red eye on the BlackBerry is more intrusive than you might think. If your phone is by the bed, you are highly likely to check your e-mails before you go to bed and also first thing when you wake up. Notice how it affects your thoughts and feelings. Pay attention to this behavior and its consequences, and if they are not positive, remind yourself you can do something about it.

- If you have trouble falling asleep, taking a hot bath about an hour and half before you want to go to bed may help. As the body temperature cools, we feel sleepier.

- Keep the bedroom for sleeping and avoid watching television, working on your laptop or tablet. Give your brain a rest for a reasonable period of time before you want to sleep.

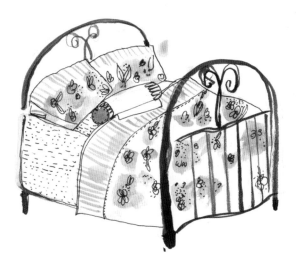

Breathing Through the Body

In a half-awake state, you may not be alert enough to judge what practice to choose or how to do it. The following is perfect for just that state of semi-consciousness and can also be done while wide-awake. Doing this will help you tune into your body more quickly and easily, and when we focus our attention on the body we are disengaging from our thoughts. If we do this when are still half asleep we are more likely to keep our thinking mind at bay.

PRACTICE TWO

★ Lie flat on your back and imagine that you are breathing in through the soles of your feet. As you breathe in, the breath travels up the legs and through the torso and as the in-breath turns into an out-breath, you are breathing out through the crown of the head. Continue in this way for as long as you wish.

★ I find it easier to breathe in through the feet and out through the top of the head but it doesn't really matter, so breathe in whichever direction feels right for you. What we are doing is allowing the breath to sweep through the body in a regular rhythm, entering and exiting the body.

★ Remember that we are not doing this in order to fall asleep. If you do, that's a bonus, but it is important to let go of that expectation otherwise every second or so you will jump out of the body and back into your head, measuring how sleepy you are (or not) and judging the experience. This is what we are trying to let go of.

Counting Breaths

Counting sheep is a time-honored way to fall asleep, but I find there is always a risk of getting too invested in the sheep. I start thinking about the landscape—if it's winter I worry about the sheep freezing in the snow, or perhaps it's spring and then there are all those lambs to count, twins and triplets, and that one has got separated from its mother... I don't know how many sheep there are in the first place so I have no idea when I've lost count and where to start again and I quickly get tangled up in thinking. Whatever object we choose to focus on, the mind will often come up with inventive ways to distract us. We can minimize this by bringing two techniques together—counting and turning our attention to the body. We can do this by counting breaths.

PRACTICE THREE

Find the place where you can feel the physical sensation of breathing most strongly, commonly the belly, the chest, or around the nostrils/upper lip. It might be helpful you can place your hands on the belly.

As you breathe in, count one, breathe out. On the next in-breath, count two, and so on.

Continue counting up to ten and then start again at one. If you go past ten, at the moment of realization, simply break off and return to one. You will often go past ten. Remember that we are practicing bringing the wandering mind back, so the more we do this, the greater the exercise we are giving that "muscle of awareness."

The neural pathways for thought and exploring physical sensations are the same, so the body can only do one at any one time. Although our mind will always wander, we are making it harder by focusing on a bodily sensation rather than a thought such as sheep. We use a limited count so we know when we have wandered away and where to come back to.

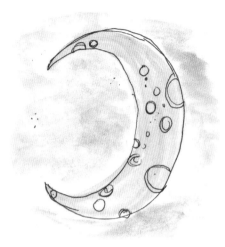

DEEP SLEEP

Yoga nidra is the centuries-old yoga practice of deep sleep. It can be quite a long practice, of about 45–50 minutes in length, and I find that if I listen to a guided yoga nidra, I sleep more deeply and wake earlier, feeling more rested. It is easiest done listening to someone guiding you. There are numerous recordings available on the Internet for free or to buy (see page 140). The following practice follows the same principles as yoga nidra. It is simple to follow and thus easy to remember, so if you can grasp the basic principles, it is something you can do without relying on any external devices. I find the visualization easier while lying down, but you can also do this as a sitting practice.

Remember that when we do this practice the order in which you do it does not matter. **We are simply moving our attention around the body**—focusing our attention on a particular area and then widening our awareness to include the whole body. You can repeat sections or the whole thing several times. You may or may not fall asleep, so it is important to practice without expecting a particular outcome.

TRY THIS

....

★ Lie on your back, with your arms and legs outstretched, feet falling apart, and the hands a little away from the body. Take a few moments to connect with the body by lightly focusing your attention on the breath.

★ Become aware of the **right side of the body**. Bring the right side of the body into awareness: the right foot, leg, arm, and torso, all of it.

★ Let go of the right side of the body and, in your mind's eye, bring the l**eft side of the body** into awareness: the left foot, leg, arm, and torso. Picture the whole of the left side of the body.

★ Let go of the left side of the body and, for a minute or two, become aware of the **entire body**, from the toes to the top of the head, from the tips of the fingers to the length of the back, hold the complete body in awareness.

★ Now let go of the complete body, become aware only of the **body below the waist**. In your mind's eye, become aware of the feet—the heel, sole, and toes of each foot—and the lower legs, knees, thighs, buttocks, pelvis, and belly. Hold the lower half of the body in awareness.

★ Let go of the lower half of the body and become aware of the **top half of the body**—the area above the waist: the back, shoulders, arms, and hands, the back of the neck and the head. Hold the top half of the body in awareness.

★ Let go of the top half of the body and become aware of the **entire body** lying here.

★ Now imagine that the body has been segmented horizontally, becoming aware of the **back of the body**, the area that is in contact with the bed or floor. Move your attention around and notice the points of contact or the absence of contact.

★ Let go of the back of the body, become aware of the **front of the body**. Imagine the area above that horizontal midline—the face, the chest, the belly, the front of the thighs, and shins.

★ Let go of the front of the body, become aware of the **entire body**—the torso, the limbs, the front, back, and sides. **Rest with the entire body in awareness.**

WHERE TO GO NEXT

This book can only give an introduction to mindfulness and if it is something that interests you I strongly recommend you look for a course near you. There are many different types of group available where individuals can learn how to establish their own mindfulness practice. I run courses in the UK and you can find out more at my website www.mindfulness-meditation-now.com. The Be Mindful website http://bemindful.co.uk has a UK-wide course locator.

Centers of expertise in the UK include:

Centre for Mindfulness Research and Practice in North Wales at www.bangor.ac.uk/mindfulness

Oxford Centre for Mindfulness https://oxfordmindfulness.org

For more information on mindfulness in Scotland www.mindfulnessscotland.org.uk

In the USA, the Center for Mindfulness www.umassmed.edu/cfm/index.aspx runs various leadership and workplace programmes as well as courses for individuals. The site also has a list of trained practitioners.

To download guided yoga nidra meditation (see page 138) go to www.yoganidranetwork.org/downloads

There are too many good books on mindfulness out there to list here—some are very academic and others aimed more at the general reader, some are by practicing Buddhists but others are more secular in nature. Authors I particularly recommend are Mark Williams, Jon Kabat-Zinn, Pema Chodron, Sharon Salzberg, Jack Kornfield, Joseph Goldstein, and Thich Nhat Hahn. Further reading specifically on mindfulness in the workplace is listed opposite.

FURTHER READING

If you would like to read more about using mindfulness in the workplace or the research behind it, the following books or articles might be helpful.

Adams, Juliet, "The business case for mindfulness in the workplace", www.mindfulnet.org, January 2012 This website has useful information on research and examples of introducing and using mindfulness in the workplace.

Carroll, Michael, *Awake at Work*, Shambhala, 2004

Chaskalson, Michael, *The Mindful Workplace*, Wiley-Blackwell, 2011

Chodron, Pema, *Taking the Leap*, Shambala, 2010

Creswell, J.K., Baldwin, M.A., Way, M., Eisenberger, N.I., and Lieberman, M.D., "Neural Correlates of Dispositional Mindfulness During Affect Labeling" in *Psychosomatic Medicine* 69, 2007

Csikszentmihalyi, Mihaly, *Flow: The Psychology of Happiness*, Rider, 2002

Frederickson, B.L, Cohn, M.A, Coffey, K.A, Pek, J, and Finkel, S.M., "Open Hearts Build Lives: " in *Journal of Personality and Social Psychology* 95, 2008

Goleman, Daniel, *What Makes a Leader*, More than Sound, 2014
—*Focus, the Hidden Driver of Excellence*, Bloomsbury, 2013

Hanh, Thich Nhat, *Work: How to Find Joy and Meaning in Each Hour of the Day*, Parallax Press, 2012

Hanson, Rick, *Buddha's Brain: The Practical Neuroscience of Happiness, Love, and Wisdom*, New Harbinger, 2009

Kabat-Zinn, Jon, *Full Catastrophe Living*, Piatkus, 1990

Lazar, S.W., Kerr, C.E., Wasserman R.H., et al., "Meditation Experience is Associated with Increased Cortical Thickness," in *Neuroreport* 16, 2005

Mental Health Foundation, Mindfulness Report 2010

Rock, David, *Your Brain at Work*, Collins Business, 2009

Williams, Mark et al., *The Mindful Way through Depression*, Guilford Press, 2007

INDEX

ACKNOWLEDGMENTS

Many people have helped bring this book to fruition. Not least the generations of teachers who have shared their knowledge and experience of mindfulness meditation with such generosity and wisdom in numerous book and teachings. I would like to thank Cindy Richards and Lauren Mulholland, and the fabulous team at CICO books for their continued support and enthusiasm for mindfulness. Amy Louise Evans for doing such a great job (again) with illustrating a difficult subject. Professionally and personally there are a raft of people who have supported me in so many different ways, in particular Catherine Grey, Eluned Gold and the team from the Centre for Mindfulness Research and Practice at Bangor, Melissa Blacker and David Rynick, plus all my family and friends, particularly Pip and the WTs. Not forgetting those participants on my courses who over the years have taught me so much and generously shared their stories and experience of mindfulness—I continually learn so much from you. Thank you!

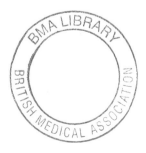

Pirates

If you enjoy PIRATES, you'll love...

SPOOKS
MONSTERS
VAMPIRES
WITCHES
SCHOOL

All published in this series by
Collins Children's Books.

PIRATES was first published in Great Britain
in 1987 by William Collins Sons & Co Ltd
First published in this format in 1995 by
HarperCollins Publishers Ltd, 77-85 Fulham Palace Road,
Hammersmith, London, W6 8JB
1 3 5 7 9 10 8 6 4 2
Text copyright © Colin and Jacqui Hawkins 1987
Illustrations copyright © Colin Hawkins 1987
The authors assert the moral right to be
identified as the authors of the work.
ISBN: 0 00 198169 2
This book is set in Galliard 12/16
Printed in Italy

Pirates

Colin and Jacqui Hawkins.

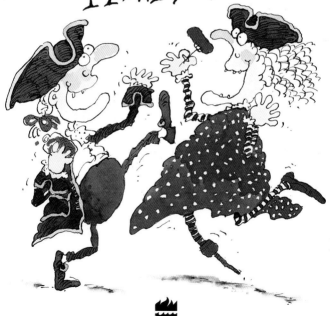

Collins

An Imprint of HarperCollinsPublishers

Pirate Spotting

Pirates are the scourge of the seven seas and the terror and dread of all honest sea-faring folk. These wicked and wily robbers, these outlaws of the oceans, are feared by friend and foe alike.

Never trust a pirate. Blink for a moment and they'll have the rings off your fingers and the bus pass from your purse. They will stop at nothing in their fierce quest for golden goodies and silver sparklies. These rum-reeking rogues will spit in your eye for a penny.

PIRATE: Who gave you that black eye?

OLD SEA DOG: Nobody, I had to fight for it.

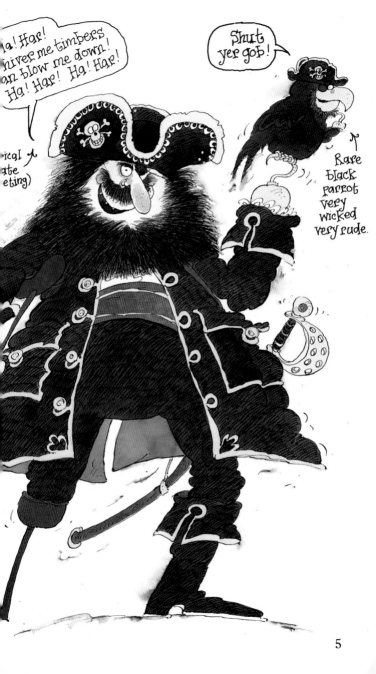

5

Can you recognise a pirate?

Would you spot one in a crowd?

If you have never seen a sea dog read carefully this old pirate lore:

"Knows't a pirate by the hook on his arm, the parrot on his shoulder and the black patch on his eye. Or 'arken to the thud clump, thud clump of his peg leg and crutch as he crosses ye olde tavern floor.

There may be a pirate in your area. Has anyone YOU know lost a parrot?

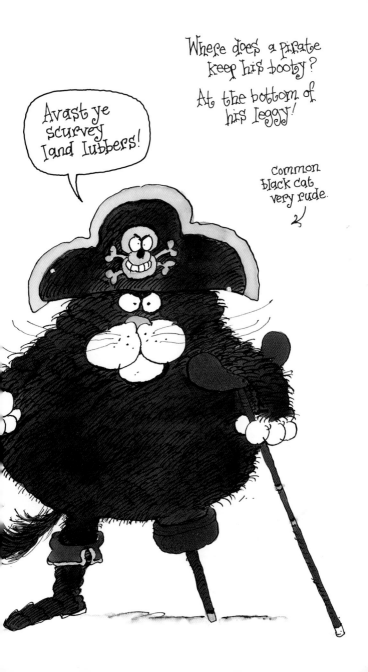

Pirat

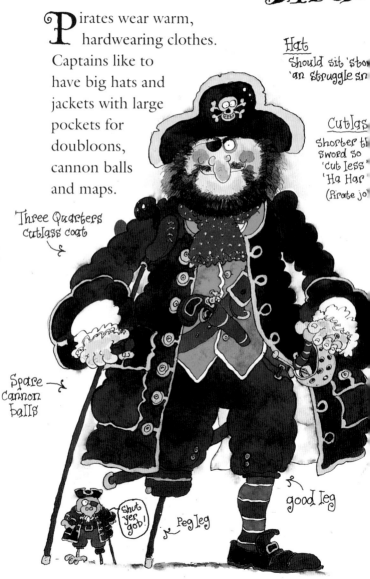

Pirates wear warm, hardwearing clothes. Captains like to have big hats and jackets with large pockets for doubloons, cannon balls and maps.

Hat
Should sit 'sho
'an struggle sn

Cutlas
Shorter th
sword so
'cut less'
'Ha Har'
(Pirate jo

Three Quarters
Cutlass coat

Spare
cannon
balls

Shut yer gob!

Peg leg

good leg

Gear

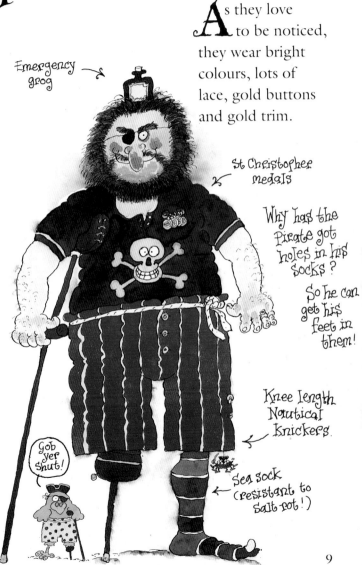

As they love to be noticed, they wear bright colours, lots of lace, gold buttons and gold trim.

Emergency grog

St Christopher medals

Why has the Pirate got holes in his socks?

So he can get his feet in them!

Knee length Nautical Knickers.

Sea sock (resistant to salt rot!)

Gob yer Shut!

Pirate Personals

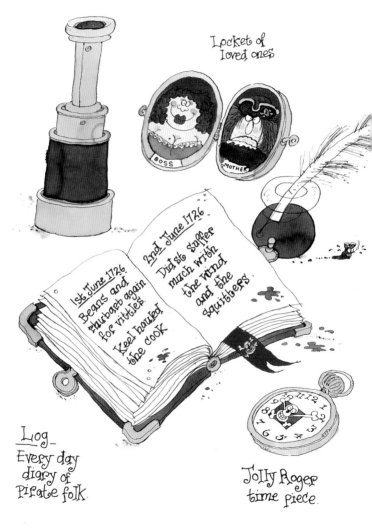

Locket of loved ones

BOSS

MOTHER

1st June 1726
Beans and rhubarb again for vittles.
Keel hauled the cook

2nd June 1726
Dids't suffer much with the wind and the squitters.

Log
Every day diary of Pirate folk.

Jolly Roger time piece.

Any pirate who still
has his teeth and
ears is considered
a sissy.

Who's that at
the door?
A pirate with
a wooden leg.
Tell him to hop it!

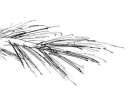

Pirates travel light. Crowded cabins and
hoards of hammocks leave little room
for pirate accessories. Life on board can be
very squashed, so the modern buccaneer has
few luxuries.

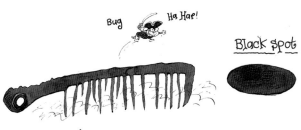

Bug   Ha Har!

Black spot to be
given to
land
lubbers
and sissys

Bug rake ↑

Black spot will
make 'ee rot.
(Old pirate curse)

Only wallies wash. Grubby pirates get clean in the sea when they fall in. No self-respecting pirate has a toothbrush – but rubs his gums and teeth (if he has any) in salt water. Long sea voyages make it difficult for those regular dental checkups, so pirates do not get the fillings they need. Pirates with problems pull out rotten teeth or spit them into the sea. Older sea rogues pride themselves on their toothless grins. It shows they've been around.

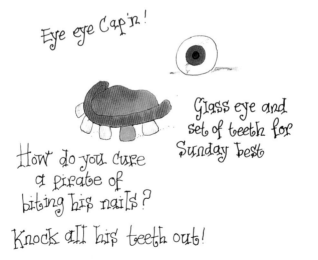

Eye eye Cap'n!

Glass eye and set of teeth for Sunday best

How do you cure a pirate of biting his nails?

Knock all his teeth out!

To the pirate who's been
sentenced to the gallows
No noose is good noose.

As it is a long way to the launderette,
pirates do not wash their clothes.
The combination of sea salt and grime
adds that extra layer they need to keep
out the cool sea breezes. Smelly seadogs
freshen up with a splash of 'Eau de Channel'.

Pirates often lose bits
of themselves in
battle, so they always
keep peg legs, hooks
and eye patches handy.

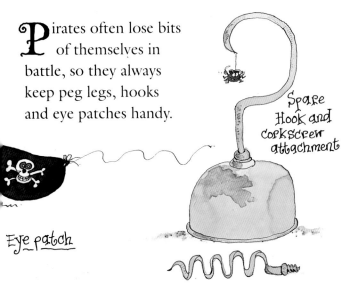

Spare
Hook and
corkscrew
attachment

Eye patch

13

Pirate Customs

Pirate crews always vote for their captain. This means anyone can be captain if they get enough votes. It is more fun being captain as you get the biggest share of the booty.

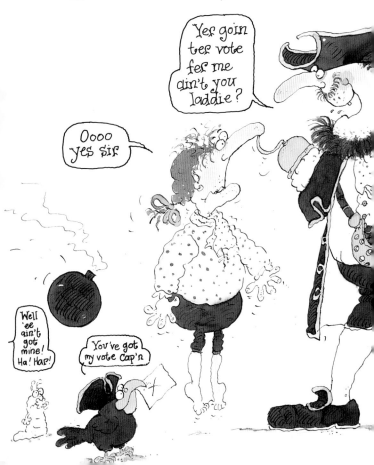

To be a successful captain you have to shout very loudly. Captains need to give orders out on deck. This can be a strain and many pirates suffer from sore throats. Some may even lose their voices completely.

Do you know of anyone with a sore throat?

Has your teacher ever lost her voice?

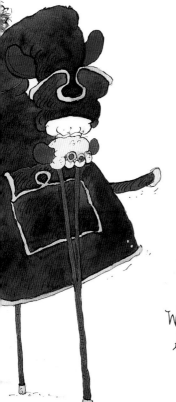

Which fish terrorises others in the sea?
Jack the kipper

Which Pirate wears the biggest hat?
The one with the biggest head.

What goes HA-HA, BONK?
A pirate laughing his head off.

On long sea voyages pirates can pass the time playing games. You may know some of these:-

Musical Hammocks
Hunt the Grog
Pass the Cannonball
Kiss Chase
Sharks (Pirates' version of Sardines)
What's the time Cap'n Hook?
Snarl (Pirates' version of Snap)

New pirates sign "the pirate's charter" and swear on the Bible to be loyal and true crew members.

Is there a Bible in your classroom?

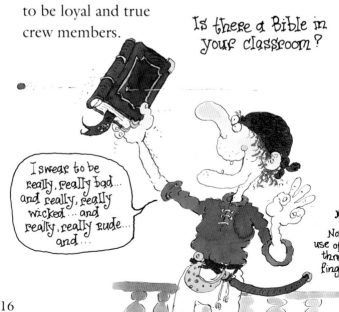

I swear to be really, really bad... and really, really wicked... and really, really rude... and...

No
use o
thre
Ring

16

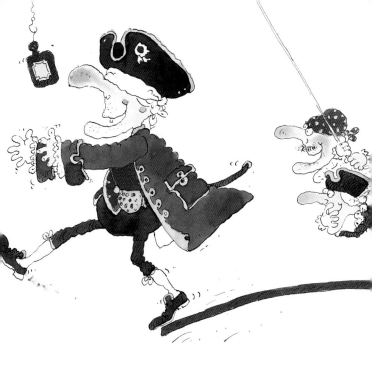

Walking the plank is a popular method of disposing of an unwanted crew member.

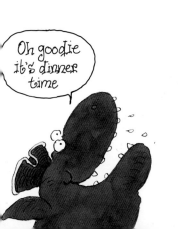

Oh goodie it's dinner time

Seven wooden planks were standing in a circle. They were having a board meeting!

17

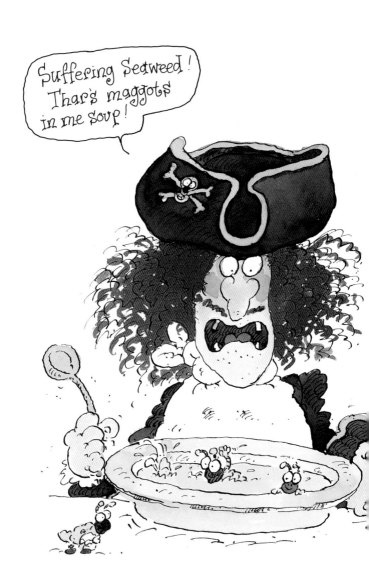

Eat up me' Hearties

Pirate food is very boring. Sea faring cooks are not usually very imaginative due to the fact that everything has gone off after a few days. Some pirate chefs, however, do have flair, and can improvise with the odd seaweed soufflé, grilled gull, poached parrot, or shark shurprise.

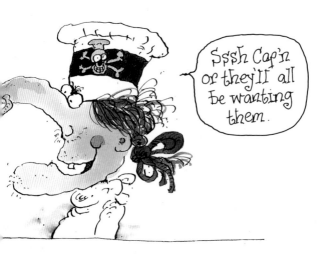

Sssh Cap'n or they'll all be wanting them.

A favourite treat is a sort of pirate muesli called Figgie Dowdie. This is a fruit pudding made with currants and raisins.

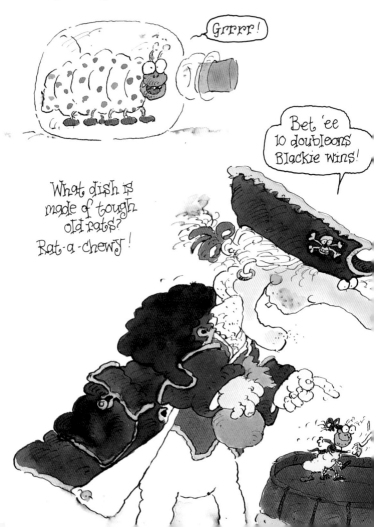

Grrrr!

Bet 'ee 10 doubleons Blackie wins!

What dish is made of tough old rats?
Rat-a-chewy!

Pirates mostly eat extremely hard biscuits called 'tack'. Unfortunately, horrible weevils and black spotted maggots like to burrow and live in these biscuits. Some pirates love maggoty tack, others dump the biscuits in their grog to improve the flavour. Hence the word 'tacky'.

Figgie Dowdie
is our favourite pud,
We get it when
we're very good.

Yer on!

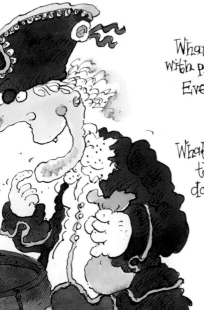

What's wrong
with pirate food?
Everything!

What did the crew of
the pirate ship
do when they
were becalmed?

Ate lots of
Baked Beans.

21

To eat hard tack
You need the knack
Or else yer pearlies
you will crack.

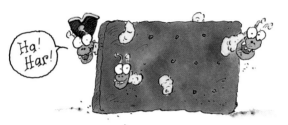

What do you do if
the cook offers
you a rock cake?

Take your pick

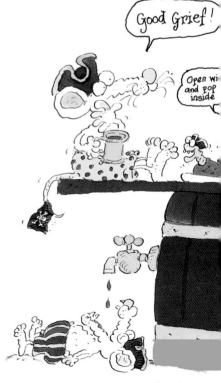

There was a pirate from Penzance
Who always wore sheet-steel pants.
He said, "Some years back
I sat down on a tack,
And I'll never again
take a chance!"

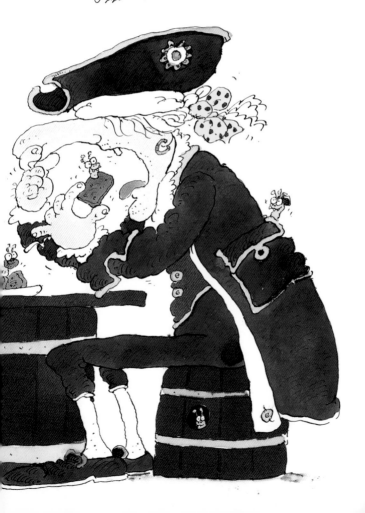

Pirate Pops

It is vital for a pirate ship to have a band on board. Singing and dancing are an important part of pirate therapy. A pirate who plays an instrument is much prized.

As evening draws in weary pirates blink blearily into the flickering lamplight, and hanging in hammocks, hum happily as the accordionist plays. Many a sea shanty can be heard wafting over the moonlit waves on a still night. Pirates need to unwind from sea stress.

What do sea monsters
like to eat?
Fish and ships!

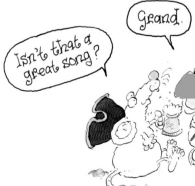

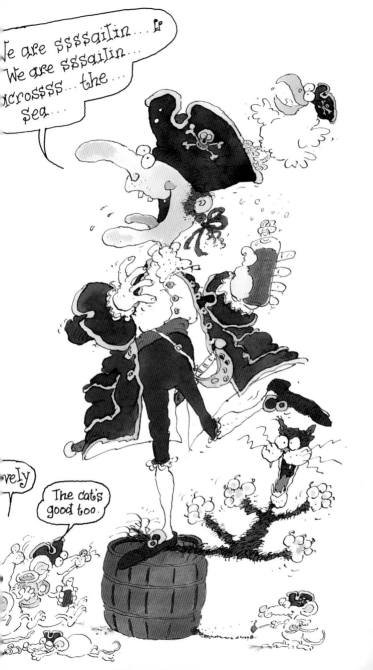

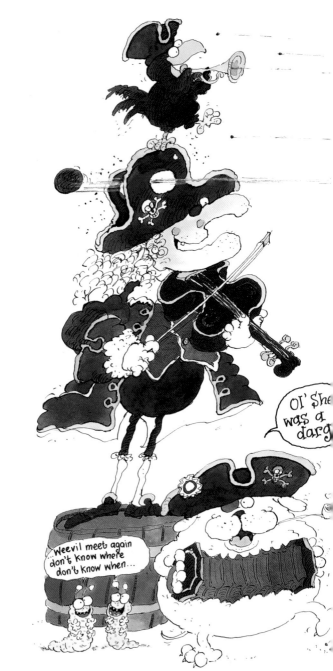

Shut yer gob!

Another function of the band is to play loudly as the pirates go into battle. The awful banging of the drums, piercing screech of the violins and the yowling of the crew, strike terror into the hearts of the enemy.

Popular pirate tunes are:-

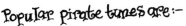

Bailing Out
It's a long way to tip a sailor
We are Assailin'
You'll never walk (the plank) Alone
  Bad Booty Blues

Wot an' 'orrible noise!

We Surrender!

No more please!

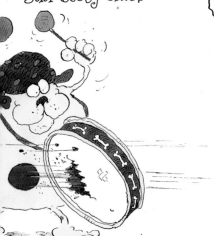

All at Sea

A pirate ship in full sail is a terrifying sight. It will send shivers to your spine and make your hair stand on end. Woe betide any God-fearing sailor when the dreaded skull and crossbones looms on the horizon.

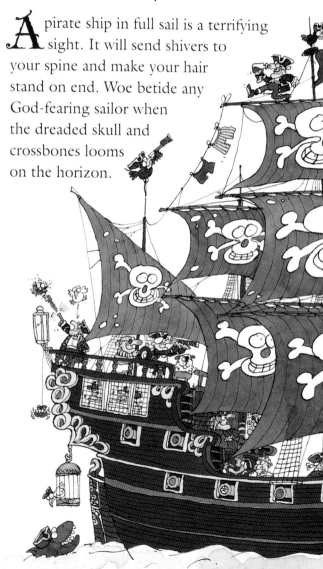

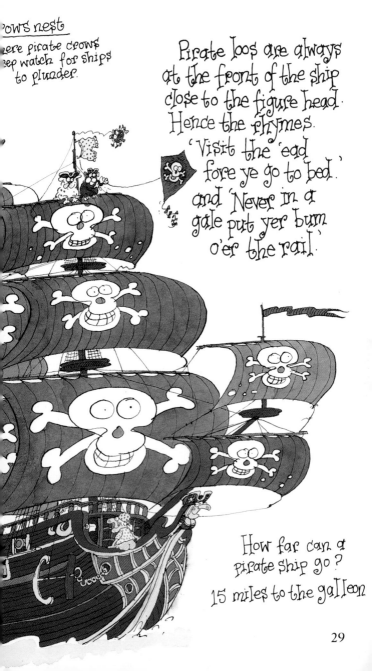

ows nest

ere pirate crows
ep watch for ships
to plunder.

Pirate loos are always
at the front of the ship
close to the figure head.
Hence the rhymes.
'Visit the 'ead
fore ye go to bed.'
and 'Never in a
gale put yer bum
o'er the rail.'

How far can a
pirate ship go?
15 miles to the galleon

29

Pirate Ploys

In order to catch and plunder treasure galleons, pirate ships have to sail very quickly. This means they have a large crew to man all the guns and keep the ships in good repair.

Pirate weather Lore

Blue patch in the sky good weather bye an bye.

Sun afore seven storm afore eleven.

Gulls on the sail watch out for the gale.

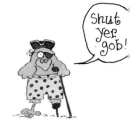

Shut yer gob!

Why did the parrot wear a raincoat?

So he could be Pollyunsaturated!

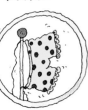

re t'is the
dy Mary out
f Dublin.

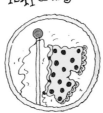

?? What's
happening?

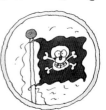

Oh! No!
T'is the Jolly Roger!

Pirates love to play tricks. One favourite pirate prank is to sneak up on treasure ships. This they do by flying the flag of honest sea-faring folk, so they can sail up close. Then, at the last moment, the wily weasels hoist the Jolly Roger and hop aboard in a flash.

What floats on the sea shouting 'Knickers'?

Crude oil!

What is the best shark repellent known to man?

The Sahara Desert!

Another pirate trick is pretending to be ladies in distress. Unsuspecting, gallant sailors hasten to rescue these helpless damsels of the seas – only to feel

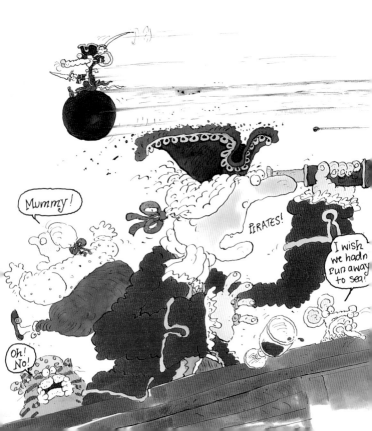

the sharp point of a cutlass in their vitals.
The sight of a great, hairy pirate in a
bonnet and petticoat will haunt many
an old sea salt to the end of his days.

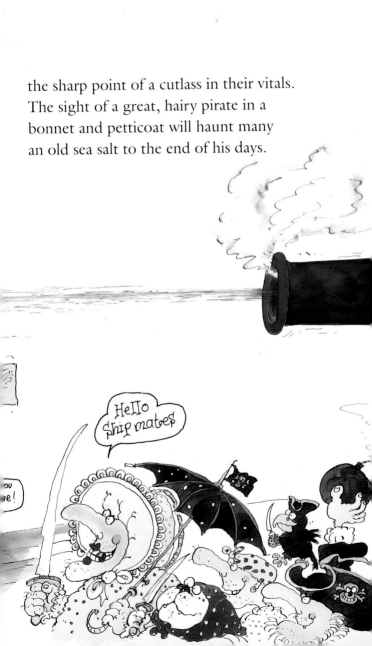

Into Battle Ha Har

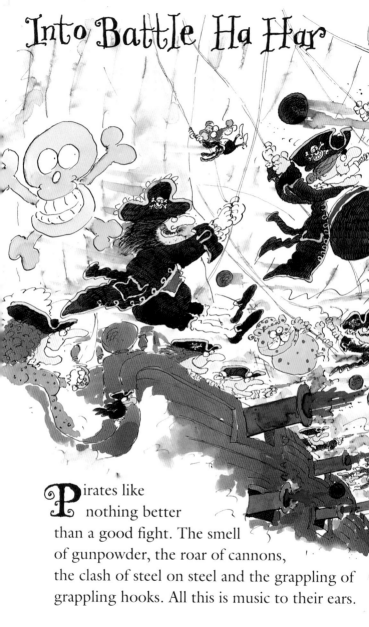

Pirates like nothing better than a good fight. The smell of gunpowder, the roar of cannons, the clash of steel on steel and the grappling of grappling hooks. All this is music to their ears.

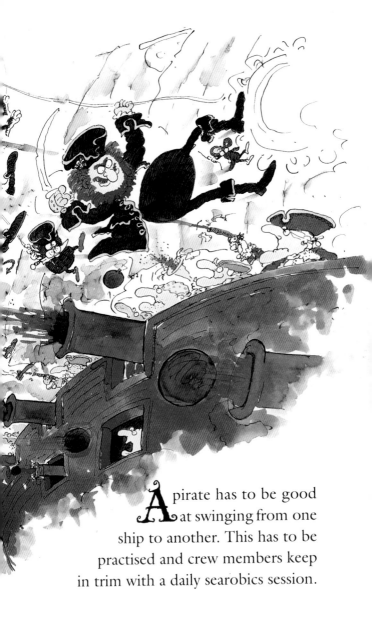

A pirate has to be good at swinging from one ship to another. This has to be practised and crew members keep in trim with a daily searobics session.

Treasure Island

Pirates who collect lots of treasure like to bury it on deserted islands to keep it safe. Sometimes they draw maps to help them remember where they left it. As they do daft drawings and silly spelling, pirates often cannot find the treasure when they return to dig it up. This means it is still waiting to be found.

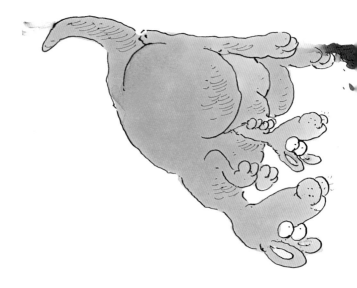

Who has 8 guns and
terrorizes the ocean?
Billy the Squid!

What do you say
to an octopus at
the dinner table?

Which fish is also
a poet?

An eel, because he
is a Longfellow.

Get your elbow,
elbow, elbow,
elbow, elbow,
elbow, elbow,
elbow off the table!

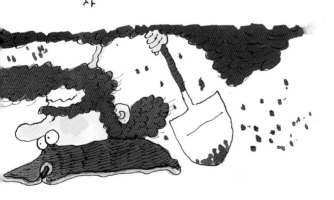

In their search for buried treasure,
pirates become enthusiastic diggers.

What's an Octopus?
An eight-sided cat!

What do you get if you cross a parrot and an elephant?

Something that tells everything it remembers.

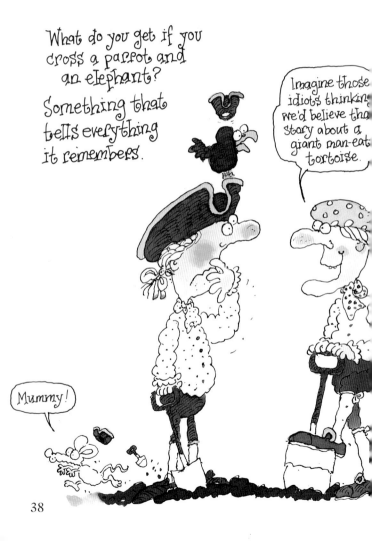

Imagine those idiots thinking we'd believe that story about a giant man-eating tortoise.

Mummy!

Long ago the island of Tortuga was a hot favourite with pirates. Rumour has it that a huge hoard of treasure is still there, guarded by a giant tortoise called Tommy.

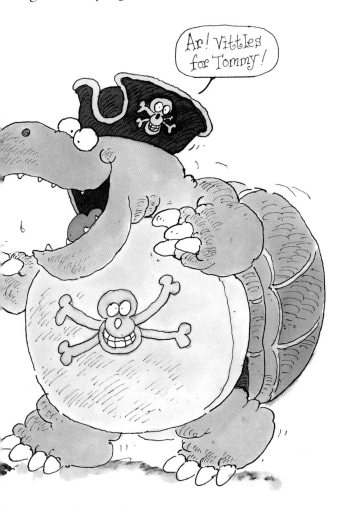

Pirate captains can be very greedy and take twice as much treasure as everyone else. Some captains (especially those with one eye) are not very good at counting, so they do not divide the spoils equally. This can make them unpopular with the crew!

What do you call a Scottish parrot?
A macaw.

Where does a 3 ton parrot sleep?
Anywhere it wants to!

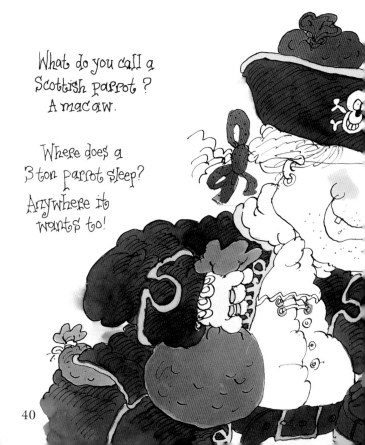

Advertisement in
The Pirate Post:

LOST: Green parrot
with half its tail
missing. Chipped
beak. Blind in one
eye. Limps a bit.
Answers to the
name LUCKY.

What does a pirate
feed his parrot?
Polyfiller!

Why is that parrot green?
It's not ripe yet.

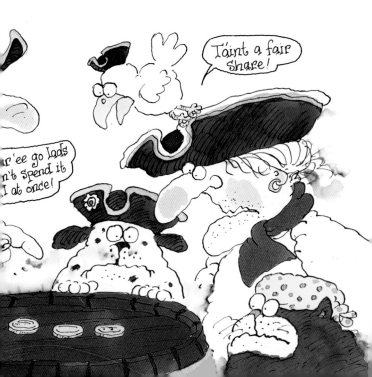

Pirates in Petticoats

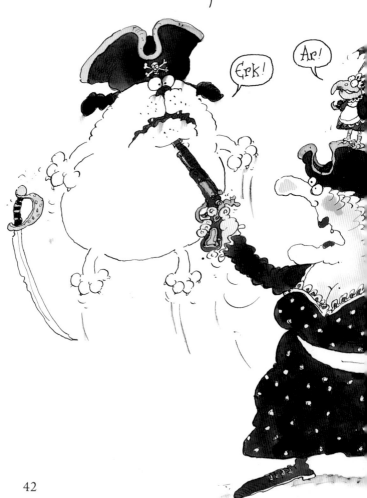

nne Bonney and Mary Read were notorious lady pirates of days gone by. These hellcats of the oceans were a fearsome pair, who struck terror in the hearts of their crew. They were particularly fierce if a pirate was not polite and forgot to say "please" and "thank you".

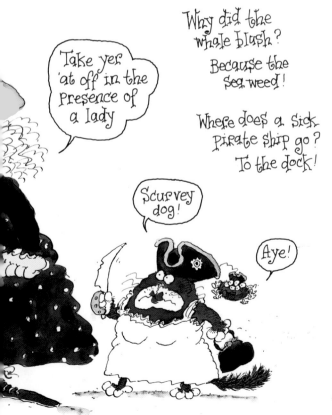

Why did the whale blush?
Because the sea weed!

Where does a sick pirate ship go?
To the dock!

Take yer 'at off in the presence of a lady

Scurvey dog!

Aye!

M any mums today like a spin on the high seas.
Perhaps your mum is a lady pirate.

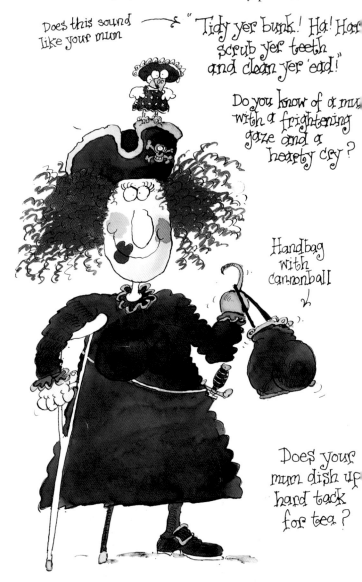

Does this sound
like your mum

"Tidy yer bunk! Ha! Ha!
scrub yer teeth
and clean yer 'ead!"

Do you know of a mum
with a frightening
gaze and a
hearty cry?

Handbag
with
cannonball

Does your
mum dish up
hard tack
for tea?

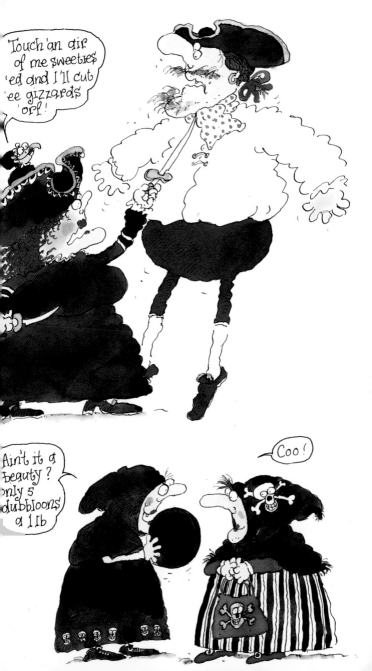

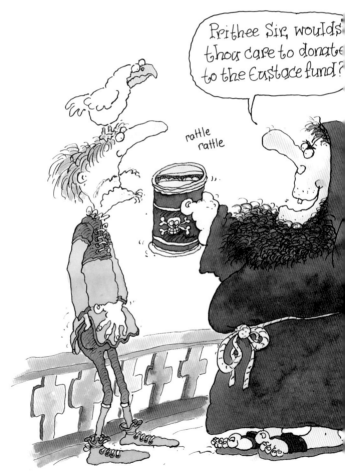

Eustace the Monk

A 12th century pirate known as the 'Black Monk'. People said he had magic powers and could make his ship invisible. It was certainly difficult to cross the Channel without giving him a donation.

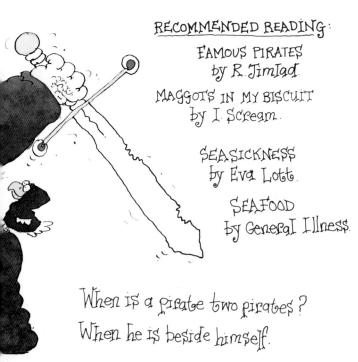

RECOMMENDED READING:

FAMOUS PIRATES
by R. Jimlad.

MAGGOTS IN MY BISCUIT
by I. Scream.

SEASICKNESS
by Eva Lott.

SEAFOOD
by General Illness.

When is a pirate two pirates?
When he is beside himself.

Who's Who

Chin Yin and Hsi Kai

Two notorious Chinese pirates, who held a British crew hostage for a huge ransom. This cunning Eastern pair spotted the shiny, brass buttons on the officers' uniforms. Thinking they were gold, they naturally presumed the English navy was very rich. They were wong.

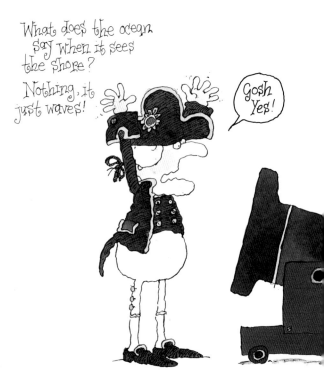

What does the ocean say when it sees the shore?

Nothing, it just waves!

Gosh Yes!

What lies at the bottom
of the sea and shivers?
A nervous wreck.

Why does the
ocean roar?
Because it has
crabs on its
bottom!

What sea creatures
are always lazy?
Oysters, because they
are always found in beds!

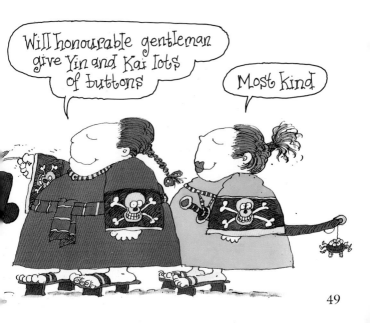

Will honourable gentleman
give Yin and Kai lots
of buttons

Most kind

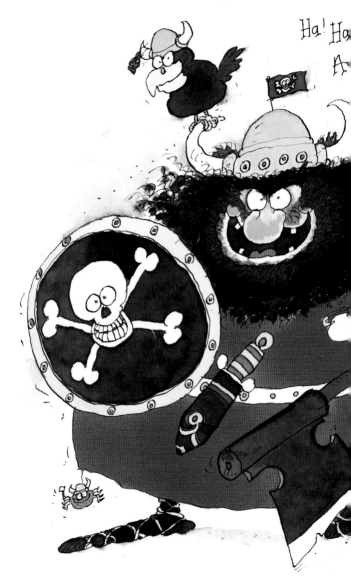

Ha! Ha
A

Olaf the Viking

One of the earliest pirates. This chap thought he was very funny, and his gruesome giggling and loony laughter warned enemies of his approach.

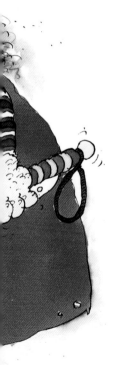

ay
!
Har!

What happened to the man with two wooden legs when his trousers caught fire?
He was burnt to the ground.

Why is it easy to fool a shark?
They'll swallow anything!

Even More Who's Who

Blackbeard (Edward Teach)

One of the most fearsome looking pirates of all times. Blackbeard was extremely hairy, with an enormous black beard and hairy hands. His favourite trick was to go into battle with lighted tapers flaming in his beard.

Avast! and Belay! or I'll cut 'ee gizzerds orf!

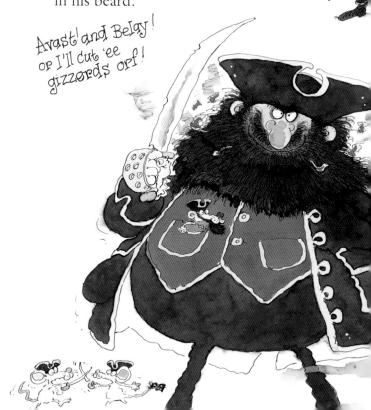

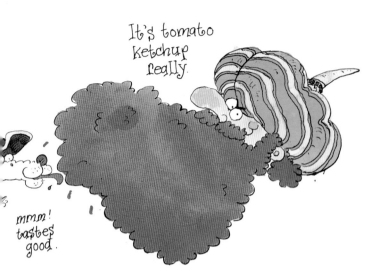

It's tomato ketchup really.

mmm! tastes good.

Barbarossa (Redbeard)

This pest of a pirate plundered the coasts of France and Spain. Some people said that he dyed his beard with the blood of his enemies.

How do you make a tall pirate short?

Get him to lend you all his money.

Ali Pasha

An evil and vicious Eastern pirate who killed or enslaved Christians. People often thought he kept his treasure in his turban!

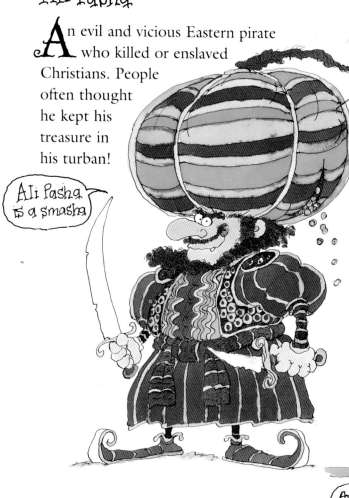

Ali Pasha is a smasha

Why can't you play
cards on a ship?
Because the captain
keeps standing
on the deck.

Bartholomew Roberts

A very strict pirate who made all his
crew members be in their hammocks
by eight o'clock. On Sundays he read the
Bible to his crew, and never drank anything
other than tea.

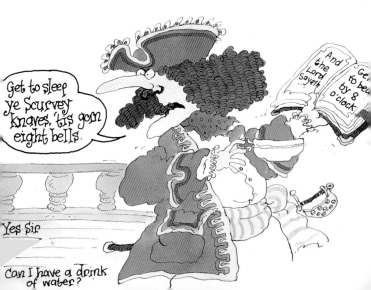

Pirate Yarn

There was an old sea dog
Who loved to drink plenty
   of grog.

At the Mad Maggot's Bar
He told tales of afar
And of ships that got lost
   in the fog.

With his eye on a wench
He'd sit on a bench
   His yarns they were
      awfully scarey...

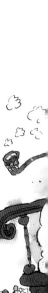

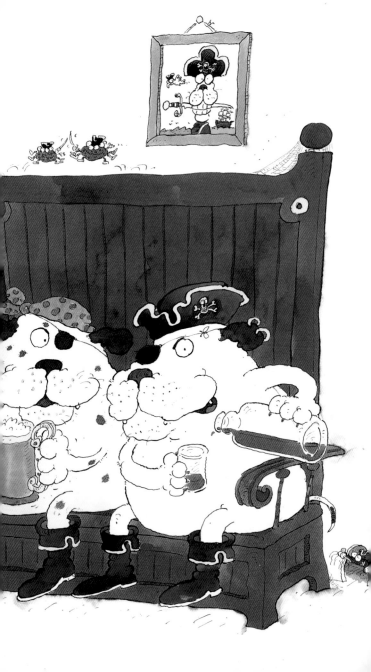

... Of terrible gales
Or 'orrid great whales
and creatures who looked
very hairy!

"The places I've been
And the booty I've seen
You folks would not
think it true."

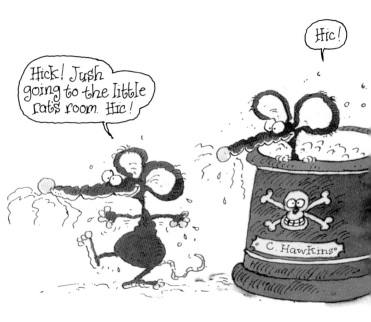

"With cutlass and sword
  We'd throw men overboard
And capture the captain and crew!"

At the end of the day
This pirate would say
That rovin' it gave him
   no pleasure,

But as the dawn broke
  And the sea dog awoke,
He'd set sail to look for
   more treasure.
Ha Har!

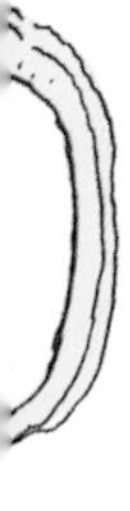

Why did the
old sea dog wear
    black boots?
His brown ones
were at the menders.

At the end of every adventure,
pirates love to throw a party.
Swilling much grog and munching
burnt, black sausages, they dance
and sing till dawn.

The best place for a party
on board ship is where
the funnel be!

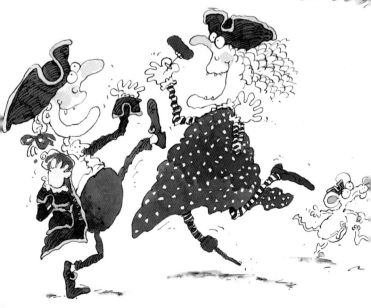

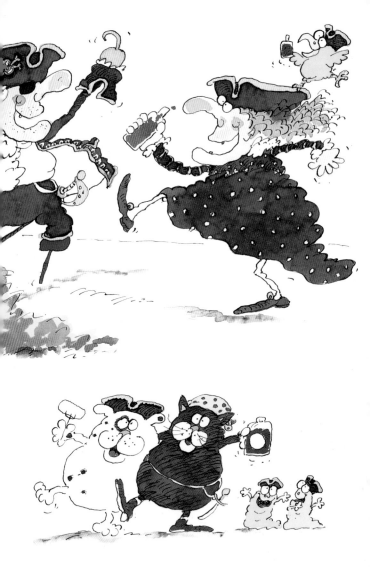

"Yo, ho, ho and
a bottle of rum,
A burnt, black
sausage in my tum.
So put on your peg leg,
Yer eye-patch too,
If you're after treasure
you can join our crew."

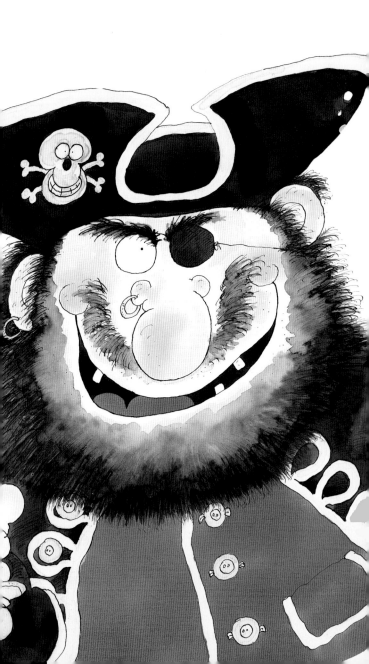

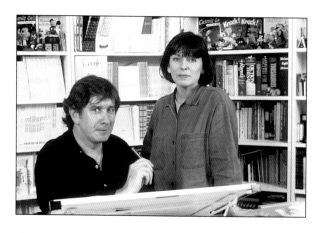

COLIN AND JACQUI HAWKINS create wonderful books together. As they each do both the writing and the illustrating, the way they work is a mysterious secret. As Colin says: "What's spooky is that when we are not together it doesn't work, and spookier still is that when neither of us are there...nothing happens! The nearest analogy is a visually-creative, brilliantly-talented scriptwriting team of two."

Colin was born in Blackpool and Jacqui in Oxford and they both studied illustration. They now live in Blackheath, London, and have two children, Finbar and Sally. When they used to read to their children, Colin and Jacqui would add their own jokes and humour to the stories. This desire to make children's books funnier, together with their talent for illustrating, led them into their current occupation. The first book they had published was WITCHES and since then Colin and Jacqui Hawkins have become two of the best-known names in the world of children's books.